Small Animal Ear Diseases

Small Animal Ear Diseases

An Illustrated Guide

Louis N. Gotthelf, DVM

Animal Hospital of Montgomery
Montgomery, Alabama

W.B. SAUNDERS COMPANY
A Harcourt Health Sciences Company

Philadelphia   London   Toronto   Sydney

W.B. SAUNDERS COMPANY
A Harcourt Health Sciences Company

The Curtis Center
Independence Square West
Philadelphia, Pennsylvania 19106

Library of Congress Cataloging-in-Publication Data

Gotthelf, Louis N.

Small animal ear diseases : an illustrated guide / Louis N.
Gotthelf.—1st ed.

p.   cm.

ISBN 0–7216–7750–9

1. Dogs—Diseases.   2. Cats—Diseases.   3. Ear—Diseases.
   4. Otitis in animals.   I. Title.

SF992.074G68   2000636.7′08978—dc21   99–40018

Editor-in-Chief: Lisette Bralow
Acquisitions Editor: Raymond R. Kersey
Project Manager: Edna Dick
Production Manager: Pete Faber
Illustration Specialist: Peg Shaw

SMALL ANIMAL EAR DISEASES: An Illustrated Guide   ISBN 0–7216–7750–9

Printed in the United States of America.

Last digit is the print number: 9   8   7   6   5   4   3   2   1

Contributors

Margo Ruth Roman-Auerhahn, BS, DVM
Staff Clinician and Owner Veterinarian, MASH Main St Animal
Services of Hopkinton, Hopkinton, Massachusetts
Anatomy of the Canine and Feline Ear

**Lisa J. Forrest, VMD, Diplomate American College of Veterinary
Radiology**
Clinical Associate Professor, Radiology, University of Wisconsin, Madison
School of Veterinary Medicine, Madison, Wisconsin
Advanced Imaging Techniques

Louis N. Gotthelf, DVM
Animal Hospital of Montgomery, Montgomery, Alabama
*Examination of the External Ear Canal; Factors That Predispose the Ear to Otitis Externa;
Inflammatory Polyps; Primary Causes of Ear Disease; Factors That Perpetuate Otitis
Externa; Otitis Media; Failure of Epithelial Migration: Ceruminoliths; Healing of the
Ruptured Eardrum*

Michael Groh, DVM
Animal Allergy and Dermatology Clinic, Lee's Summit, Missouri
Allergic Otitis Externa

**Gregg Kortz, DVM, Diplomate American College of Veterinary
Internal Medicine (Neurology)**
Adjunct Clinical Professor, Department of Surgery and Radiology, School
of Veterinary Medicine, University of California, Davis, California
Advanced Imaging Techniques

A. Kumar, BVSc, MVSc, MS, PhD

Professor, Department of Biomedical Sciences; Course Director, Small and Large Animal Gross Anatomy; Co-director, Clinical Anatomy; Tufts University School of Veterinary Medicine, North Grafton, Massachusetts
Anatomy of the Canine and Feline Ear

Philip D. Mansfield, DVM, Diplomate American Board of Veterinary Practice

Associate Professor, Department of Small Animal Surgery and Medicine, College of Veterinary Medicine, Auburn University, Auburn, Alabama
Ototoxicity of Topical Preparations

Steven A. Melman, VMD

Founder, DermaPet Animal Behavior and Dermatology Clinic, Potomac, Maryland and Palm Springs, California
Diagnosis and Treatment of Pruritic Otitis

Starr C. Miller, BS, Pharmacy

Pharmacist, Department of Clinical Sciences, College of Veterinary Medicine, Nursing and Allied Health, Tuskegee University, Tuskegee, Alabama
Ototoxicity of Topical Preparations

Norma White-Weithers, MS, DVM, Diplomate American College of Veterinary Dermatology

Assistant Professor, Department of Clinical Sciences, Tuskegee University School of Veterinary Medicine; Tuskegee Institute, Tuskegee, Alabama
Ceruminous Otitis Externa

Ronald E. Whitford, DVM

Chief of Staff, Animal Clinic of North Clarksville, Clarksville, Tennessee
Marketing Ear Care and Otitis Therapy: The Nuts and Bolts

Preface

I have been a practicing veterinarian in small animal practice for 20 years and I am keenly aware of the variety of visual reference books available to practitioners. As veterinarians, we rely on these references to help us recognize diseases that we have learned about but never have seen firsthand in our practices. Adequate reference material has become an indispensable part of our veterinary practices.

Ear disease occurs commonly and is well recognized by every veterinarian. Recognition of disease is one thing; effectively treating otitis is quite another. Most practitioners encounter several cases of ear disease weekly and also get to see dogs and cats that have shown no response to previous treatment.

Reference material on the topic of diseases of the ear is sparse in the veterinary literature, considering the number of cases of otitis externa seen. I am not aware of a single reference book devoted exclusively to ear diseases of dogs and cats, and until very recently have never seen a photograph of the normal dog's eardrum in any reference. Pictures of ear diseases are not seen in the veterinary literature.

I have been using the Video Vetscope since 1996 and have identified and documented a large number of pathological conditions of the ear canal, tympanic membrane, and middle ear. The photographs of a variety of those ear conditions along with some of the information I have gathered through the years have been assembled into this book. It is my hope that identifying specific ear diseases will make treatments more specific, ultimately leading to quicker resolution of ear disease.

LOUIS N. GOTTHELF

Acknowledgments

W riting a book requires much time and patience. For those people in my life who allowed me to be sequestered from them while writing it, I want to give thanks. Henry David Thoreau had his Walden Pond where he could think and reflect. I have my desks at my hospital and home as my refuge.

Thanks to my staff at Animal Hospital of Montgomery for allowing me to close my office door occasionally and work for a while each day without interruption. Writing required me to organize my thoughts in a quiet room before committing the words to the page.

Thanks to my wife, Penny, who often awoke in the morning alone in bed only to find me at the computer working on the manuscript. Thanks to my children, Janie, Gabe, and Joey, who had to be especially quiet in the house while I was working.

I want to especially express my thanks and gratitude to the contributing authors, who added their knowledge and expertise to this effort. With their busy daily schedules and numerous other commitments, they came through.

I would like to thank the cooperative owners of many of my patients whose ear photos are used in this book. Because they allowed me to take extra time with sedation and anesthesia in their pets, I was able to get very good photographic representations of various ear conditions.

Special thanks goes out to Ron Buck, president of MedRx, Inc., who took a chance on designing and manufacturing the Video Vetscope. Because of his vision, this book has become possible.

Contents

1

Anatomy of the Canine and Feline Ear   1
A. Kumar and Margo Ruth Roman-Auerhahn

2

Examination of the External Ear Canal   25
Louis N. Gotthelf

3

Factors That Predispose the Ear to Otitis Externa   45
Louis N. Gotthelf

4

Inflammatory Polyps   79
Louis N. Gotthelf

5

Primary Causes of Ear Disease   87
Louis N. Gotthelf

6

Factors That Perpetuate Otitis Externa   99

Louis N. Gotthelf

7

Allergic Otitis Externa   113

Michael Groh

8

Otitis Media   121

Louis N. Gotthelf

9

Ototoxicity of Topical Preparations   145

Philip D. Mansfield and Starr C. Miller

10

Failure of Epithelial Migration: Ceruminoliths   155

Louis N. Gotthelf

11

Healing of the Ruptured Eardrum   169

Louis N. Gotthelf

12

Ceruminous Otitis Externa   181

Norma White-Weithers

13

Advanced Imaging Techniques   197

Lisa J. Forrest and Gregg Kortz

14

Diagnosis and Treatment of Pruritic Otitis   213

Steven A. Melman

15

Marketing Ear Care and Otitis Therapy: The Nuts and Bolts   223
Ronald E. Whitford

Appendix
Ear Product Formulary   249

Index   253

1

Anatomy of the Canine and Feline Ear

A. Kumar, DVM, PhD
Margo Ruth Roman-Auerhahn, DVM

The basic anatomical components of the dog and cat ear are:

- Auricle or pinna
- Auditory canal or external auditory meatus
- Middle ear
- Internal ear

Structure of the External Ear

The external ear is composed of three elastic cartilages: annular, scutiform, and auricular (Fig. 1–1). The annular and auricular cartilages form

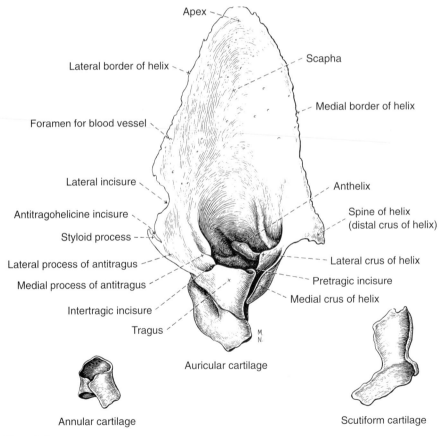

Apex

Lateral border of helix

Scapha

Medial border of helix

Foramen for blood vessel

Lateral incisure

Anthelix

Antitragohelicine incisure

Spine of helix
(distal crus of helix)

Styloid process

Lateral process of antitragus

Lateral crus of helix

Medial process of antitragus

Pretragic incisure

Intertragic incisure

Medial crus of helix

Tragus

Auricular cartilage

Annular cartilage

Scutiform cartilage

Figure 1–1

Cartilages of the right external ear. (From Evans HE (ed): Miller's Anatomy of the Dog, 3rd ed. Philadelphia, WB Saunders, 1993.)

the external ear canal, and the auricular cartilage expands to form the pinna. The scutiform cartilage lies medial to the auricular cartilage within the auricular muscles that attach to the head (Fig. 1–2).

Pinna or Auricle

The pinna or auricle is a highly visible structure. Cartilage of the pinna is breed-specific in the dog but mostly upright in the cat. It is designed to localize and collect sound waves and transmit them to the tympanic membrane (eardrum). The ear is moved by three sets of muscles (rostral, ventral, and caudal) that are innervated by branches of the facial nerve (cranial nerve VII).

The leaf-shaped pinna of the external ear is broad with medial (rostral) and lateral (caudal) margins. The caudal margin of the pinna exhibits a

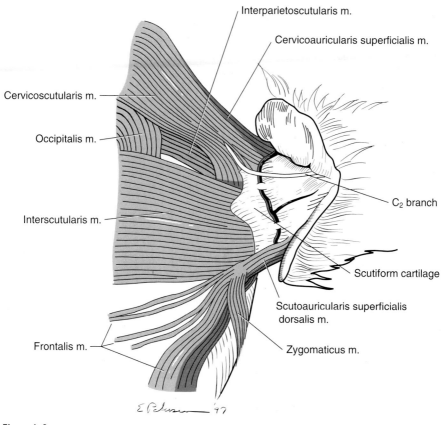

Figure 1–2

Location of the scutiform cartilage in relation to some of the external ear muscles in the dog.

cutaneous pouch called the *marginal pouch* (Fig. 1–3). This pouch has no obvious function. The skin on the concave surface of the pinna is very tightly connected to the underlying auricular cartilage, accentuating all the auricular prominences (see Fig. 1–3). The skin covering the auricular cartilage may show breed-specific pigmentation. The shape and size of the external ear vary greatly among different breeds of dogs, mainly owing to the auricular cartilage that forms the skeleton of the pinna. It is the largest cartilage of the external ear. The broad auricular cartilage has numerous holes (see Fig. 1–1), which are traversed by branches arising from the caudal auricular artery.

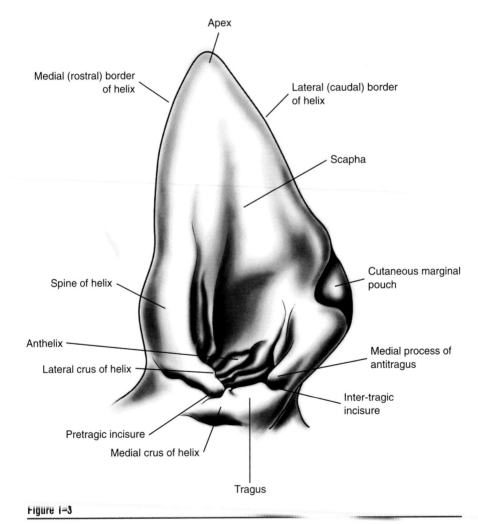

Figure 1–3

Anatomical features of the left external ear of the dog.

The auricular cartilage is broad dorsally and funnels to a narrow tube-like structure, the *tubus auris,* which fits around the annular cartilage ring. Parotid salivary gland occupies the base of the external ear, partially surrounding the tubus auris (Fig. 1–4; see also Fig. 1–5). The tubus auris encloses the vertical part of the external ear canal. The funnel-shaped cava conchae form the vertical canal and, together with the tragal, antitragal, and antihelicine borders, form the external acoustic meatus (see Fig. 1–3).

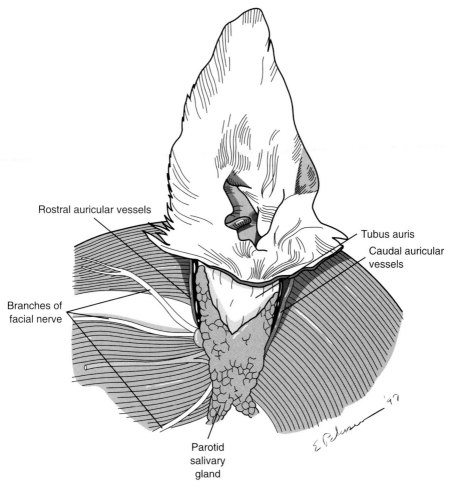

Rostral auricular vessels

Tubus auris

Caudal auricular vessels

Branches of facial nerve

Parotid salivary gland

Figure 1–4

Relationships of the tubus auris to the parotid salivary gland and auricular vessels. The facial nerve runs deep to the parotid salivary gland, immediately ventral to the annular cartilage, and gives off motor branches to the facial muscles.

Usually, entrance to the external ear canal is guarded by few fine hairs. Certain breeds, such as Airedales and Old English sheepdogs, exhibit hairy external ear canals. The external ear canal of the cat is devoid of hairs, and the ear canal is well ventilated. This may be a significant factor contributing to the lower incidence of external ear canal infections in cats. A hairy ear canal interferes with proper drainage and aeration of the canal in chronic otitis externa complicated by granulomatous lesions, leading to exacerbation of the condition.

Annular Cartilage

The annular cartilage is part of the external ear canal. The pinna, formed by the cone-shaped auricular cartilage, articulates with the annular cartilage. The annular cartilage is a ring-shaped structure attached to the bony orbit of the external acoustic meatus of the temporal bone. A tubular cartilage piece, the annular cartilage surrounds the osseous external acoustic meatus (see Fig. 1–7). It is attached to the bony rim of the external acoustic meatus by fibrous tissue that permits some degree of movement of the external ear. The annular cartilage encloses the horizontal part of the external ear canal.

Scutiform Cartilage

The scutiform cartilage is an L-shaped structure located over the temporalis muscle. It does not contribute to the formation of the external ear or its canal. The scutiform cartilage is attached to the midline raphe of the head and neck by numerous muscles (see Fig. 1–2). Muscles also extend from the scutiform cartilage to the auricular cartilage. The scutiform cartilage functions like a fulcrum, providing for efficient movement of the auricle. It can be considered to function like a sesamoid cartilage. It lies over a fat cushion (corpus adiposum auriculae) on the dorsal surface of the temporalis muscle.

Structure of the Ear Canal

The external ear canal in the dog is 5 to 10 cm long and 4 to 5 mm wide (Fig. 1–5). The ear canal consists of an initial vertical part, which may extend an inch. The vertical canal runs ventrally and slightly rostrally before bending to a shorter horizontal canal that runs medially and forms the horizontal part of external ear canal. Because the external ear is elastic, the ear canal can be straightened enough to permit otoscopic examination.

The vertical part and most of the horizontal part of the canal are cartilaginous, but the deepest part is osseous. The ear canal is lined by skin

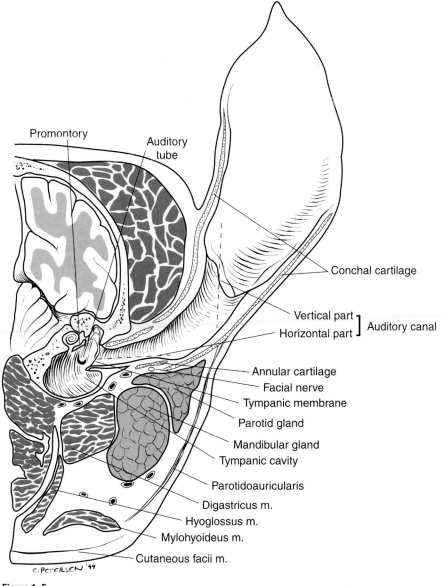

Promontory

Auditory tube

Conchal cartilage

Vertical part ⎤
Horizontal part ⎦ Auditory canal

Annular cartilage
Facial nerve
Tympanic membrane
Parotid gland
Mandibular gland
Tympanic cavity
Parotidoauricularis
Digastricus m.
Hyoglossus m.
Mylohyoideus m.
Cutaneous facii m.

E. PETERSEN '99

Figure 1–5

Structure of the ear canal. (Redrawn from Bojrab MJ: Current Techniques in Small Animal Surgery I. Philadelphia, Lea & Febiger, 1975.)

containing sebaceous and ceruminous glands and hair follicles. The ceruminous glands are modified apocrine tubular sweat glands. The combined secretions of sebaceous and ceruminous glands constitute ear wax *(cerumen)*. Cerumen (1) protects the external ear canal by immobilizing foreign objects and (2) keeps the tympanic membrane moist and pliable. The external ear canal is separated from the middle ear cavity by the semitransparent tympanic membrane.

Blood Supply to the External Ear

The external ear is generously vascularized by branches of the external carotid artery. A large caudal auricular artery arises from the external carotid artery at the base of the annular cartilage, medial to the parotid salivary gland and deep to the caudal auricular muscles. This artery gives off the lateral, intermediate, and medial auricular arteries, which pass along the convex surface of the pinna, wrapping around the helicene margins as well as penetrating the scapha and supplying the skin covering the cavum conchae. In addition to providing nourishment to the tissues of the external ear, the vascular supply to the pinna may also play a minor thermoregulatory role. Venous drainage occurs via the caudal auricular and superficial temporal veins into the maxillary vein.

CLINICAL NOTE
Violent shaking of the head by the animal may contribute to fracture of the delicate auricular cartilage, resulting in severe hemorrhage within the cartilage. The blood clot (aural hematoma) may often fill the entire concave surface of the ear, requiring surgical removal of the clot.

Nerves of the External Ear

Sensory innervation of the pinna and external ear canal is provided by four nerves: the trigeminal, facial, vagus, and second cervical.

The auriculotemporal branch of the trigeminal nerve provides sensory innervation to the skin lining the horizontal part of the ear canal and the tympanic membrane itself. This nerve also provides sensory innervation to the rostral margin of the pinna and the concave surface of the pinna close to the rostral margin and the skin over the tragus.

The facial nerve is related to the ventral surface of annular cartilage, close to the osseous external acoustic meatus. The facial nerve provides substantial sensory innervation to the concave surface of the scapha and part of the cavum conchae via the rostral, middle, and caudal internal auricular branches (Fig. 1–6). Most of the vertical along with part of the horizontal ear canal lining is supplied by the lateral internal auricular branch of the facial nerve, which may contain predominantly vagal fibers.

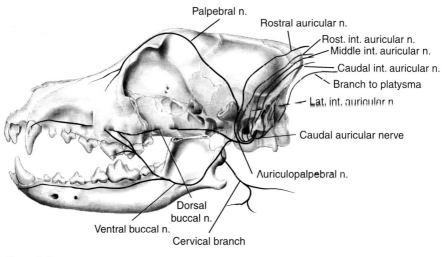

Palpebral n.
Rostral auricular n.
Rost. int. auricular n.
Middle int. auricular n.
Caudal int. auricular n.
Branch to platysma
Lat. int. auricular n
Caudal auricular nerve
Auriculopalpebral n.
Dorsal buccal n.
Ventral buccal n.
Cervical branch

Figure 1–6

Schematic drawing of sensory branches of the facial nerve that supply the external ear. Other important motor branches of the facial nerve are also shown.

Communication between the facial nerve and the vagal nerve takes place as the facial nerve exits the stylomastoid foramen (see Fig. 1–11). It is believed that these vagal branches are given off as the lateral internal auricular branch to the skin of the external ear canal. Reflex gastric vomiting may be triggered if the sensory endings of the vagus nerve are stimulated by mild ear canal irritation.

The convex surface of the pinna is provided with sensory innervation mainly by the second cervical nerve. All of the muscles of the external ear are innervated by the facial nerve.

Tympanic Membrane

The tympanic membrane (eardrum) is a thin, slightly opaque, membranous partition that separates the external ear from the middle ear. The tympanic membrane is located at a 45-degree angle in relation to the central axis of the horizontal part of the external ear canal (Fig. 1–7; see also Fig. 1–5). It is thin in the center and thicker near the periphery. The small upper portion is the *pars flaccida,* and the larger lower part is the *pars tensa* (Fig. 1–8). With the exception of the pars flaccida, the membrane is tense, being firmly attached to the surrounding bone by a fibrocartilaginous ring, the *annulus fibrocartilaginous.* This ring is attached to the osseous ring of the external acoustic meatus by fibrous tissue.

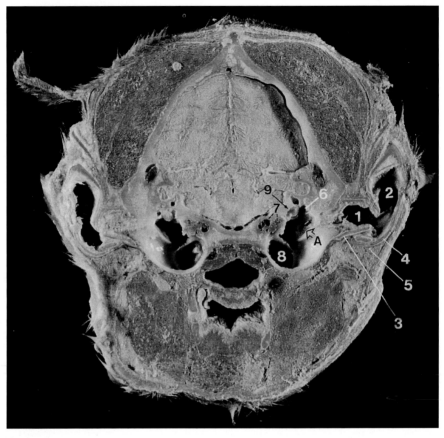

Figure 1–7

Transverse section through the head of the dog at the level of the tympanic bulla. *A*, Osseous external acoustic meatus covered by tympanic membrane. Note that the tympanic membrane is placed at an approximately 45-degree angle in relation to the central axis of the horizontal part of the ear canal. *1*, horizontal part of the ear canal; *2*, vertical part of the ear canal; *3*, annular cartilage; *4*, auricular cartilage; *5*, parotid salivary gland; *6*, epitympanic recess; *7*, carotid canal accommodating the internal carotid artery, post-ganglionic sympathetic nerves, and the ventral petrosal venous sinus (the caudal continuation of cavernous venous sinus), which drains into the internal jugular and vertebral veins; *8*, cavity of the middle ear; *9*, osseous labyrinth accommodating the internal ear.

The *pars flaccida* is a loose, opaque, pink triangular region forming the upper quadrant of the eardrum containing small branching blood vessels. Owing to its flaccid nature and rich blood supply, the pars flaccida heals rapidly if injured.

The pars tensa is thin, tough, and glistening, usually pearl-gray and translucent, although it may have opaque, radiating strands. The pars tensa, once broken, heals slowly. The external aspect of the tympanic membrane is concave because of traction on the medial surface by the manubrium of the

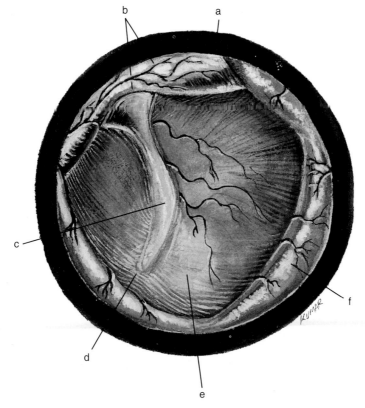

Figure 1–8

Tympanic membrane anatomy in the dog as observed through an otoscope. *a*, rim of the oto-scopic tube; *b*, flaccid part of the tympanic membrane; *c*, manubrium of malleus shining through the tympanic membrane; *d*, umbo of tympanic membrane; *e*, pars tensa of the tympanic membrane surrounding the manubrium; *f*, skin of the external acoustic meatus raised by the otoscopic tube. (Modified from DeLahunta A, Habel RE: Applied Veterinary Anatomy. Philadelphia, WB Saunders, 1986.)

malleus. The outline of the manubrium of the malleus is usually visible through the tympanic membrane as the *stria mallearis* (see Fig. 1–8).

Opposite to the distal end of the manubrium, the depressed point on the external surface of the tympanic membrane is called the *umbo membranae tympani*. The tympanic membrane is relatively thin at the center and gradually becomes thicker at its periphery, where it is attached to a rim of the annulus fibrocartilaginous.

Histologically, the tympanic membrane is made up of four layers: an external epidermal layer, an inner mucous layer, and two layers of intervening fibrous tissue. The epidermal layer is made up of a thin hairless skin consisting of a flat basal layer without any ridges and a superficial layer only a few cells thick. This stratified squamous epithelium is continuous with the epithelial lining of the external ear canal. The thin dermis contains fibroblasts and a fine vascular supply. The thicker middle fibrous layer consists of an outer layer of fibers that radiate toward the annulus fibrocartilaginous from the center of the eardrum. A layer of inner fibers are circular and are found closer to the annulus. The manubrium of the malleus is buried in the fibrous layer intercalated between the two epithelial surfaces. The arrangement of fibers in the middle layer optimizes the vibratory response of the tympanic membrane to incoming sound waves. The inner layer of the tympanic membrane is composed of a single layer of respiratory epithelium that lacks the goblet cells and cilia characteristic of respiratory epithelium. The epithelium lining the inner surface of the tympanic membrane starts as columnar at the periphery, gradually becoming cuboidal and finally squamous at the center. This layer is continuous with the mucous membrane type of respiratory epithelium covering the middle ear cavity, auditory tube, and the nasal cavity. The underlying lamina propria is thin with a fine vascular supply.

Middle Ear

The middle ear consists of the space within the osseous tympanic bulla, the opening of the auditory tube, and the three ear ossicles with their associated muscles and ligaments.

Structure of the Osseous Tympanic Bulla

It is clinically relevant to appreciate the close relationships among the facial canal, which carries the facial nerve; the petro-occipital (or carotid) canal, which carries post-ganglionic sympathetic nerves to the eye; and the periorbital structures, structures of the inner ear, and the middle ear cavity. The tympanic bulla has approximately equal dimensions (8–10 mm) in width and depth. The wall of the bulla tympanica is very thin and easy to remove.

The roof of the tympanic cavity presents a barrel-shaped prominence called the *cochlear promontory* (Figs. 1–9 and 1–10). The osseous bony cochlea is excavated within the cochlear promontory. At the caudolateral end of this promontory, a foramen called the cochlear (or round) window is located. The cochlear window is covered by a thin membrane that oscillates to dissipate vibratory energy of the perilymph in the scala tympani. Immediately lateral to the barrel-shaped promontory, a narrow vestibular (or oval) window is present, which is covered by a thin diaphragm. The footplate of the stapes is attached to the diaphragm over the vestibular window. The bony facial canal is closely related to the middle ear cavity.

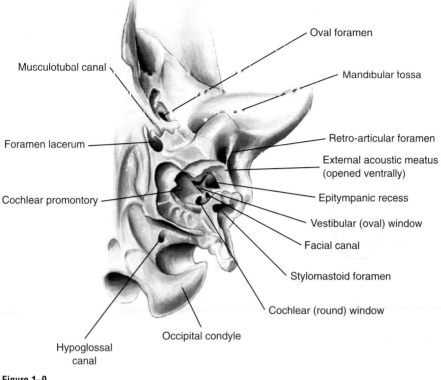

Oval foramen

Musculotubal canal

Mandibular fossa

Foramen lacerum

Retro-articular foramen

External acoustic meatus
(opened ventrally)

Cochlear promontory

Epitympanic recess

Vestibular (oval) window

Facial canal

Stylomastoid foramen

Cochlear (round) window

Hypoglossal
canal

Occipital condyle

Figure 1–9

Internal anatomy of left tympanic bulla, ventral view. The ventral wall of the bulla has been removed.

An open slit facing the vestibular window is present in the bony facial canal (see Figs. 1–9 and 1–10). This slit is the open part of the facial canal, which is covered by mucous membrane lining the tympanic bulla. The other fossae close to the external acoustic meatus accommodate the tensor tympani and stapedius muscles. The small middle ear bones, the malleus, incus, and stapes, are accommodated in an epitympanic recess located dorsal to the oval and vestibular windows, immediately medial to the opening of the external acoustic meatus.

At the caudal aspect of the tympanic bulla is a large fissure called the *tympano-occipital fissure,* which is also called the petrobasilar or petro-occipital fissure. A medial foramen in the tympano-occipital fissure that leads into a canal between the occipital and temporal bones is called the *caudal foramen lacerum.* The bony canal that extends rostrally from the caudal foramen lacerum is called the *carotid canal;* it transmits the internal carotid artery and post-ganglionic sympathetic plexus from the superior cervical ganglion (also called the carotid plexus, made up of the

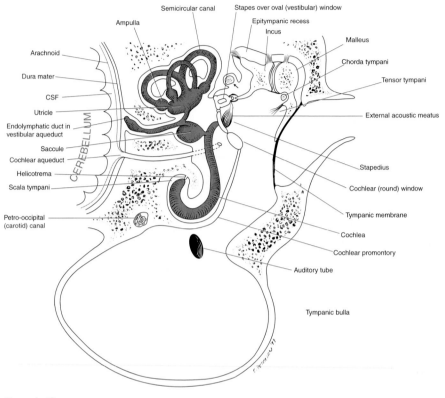

Figure 1–10

Schematic drawing of the internal and middle ear structures. The three ear ossicles form synovial joints with one another, supported by ligaments and two skeletal muscles. Note the location of the facial nerve in relation to the middle ear cavity *(arrow)*. Also shown are the relationships between subarachnoid space containing cerebrospinal fluid *(CSF)* and the inner ear via the cochlear aqueduct.

carotid nerves; Fig. 1–11). The carotid canal in its caudal extent also accommodates the ventral petrosal venous sinus (the caudal continuation of the cavernous venous sinus), which drains into the internal jugular and vertebral veins.

Ear Ossicles

The auditory ossicles—the malleus, incus, and stapes—are small movable bones that extend like a chain from the tympanic membrane and functionally connect the tympanic membrane with the vestibular (oval) window (see Fig. 1–10). The ossicles consist of compact bone formed by endochondral ossification. They form synovial joints with each other.

The malleus is the most lateral bone. It consists of a head that articulates with the incus, a thin neck, and a long manubrium, or handle. The

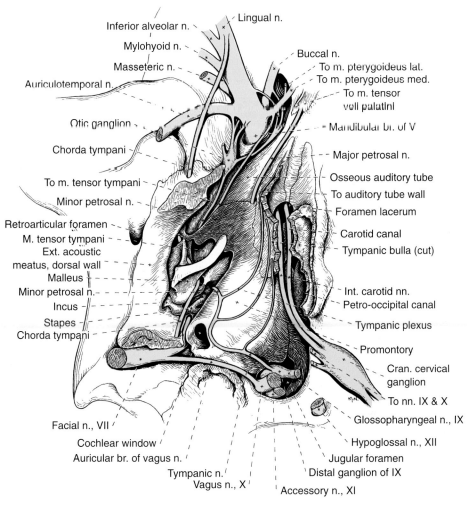

Figure 1–11

Nerves in relation to the middle ear cavity, ventral view, with most of the tympanic bulla removed. (From Evans HE (ed): Miller's Anatomy of the Dog, 3rd ed. Philadelphia, WB Saunders, 1993.)

lateral aspect of the handle is concave and is embedded in the tympanic membrane, as described earlier.

Articulating with the medial part of the incus is the stapes. It is in direct contact with the perilymph fluid through its footplate (base of stapes) attachment in the oval window.

Vibrations of the tympanic membrane are transmitted through the chain of these auditory ossicles to the perilymph fluid within the vestibule. The vestibular window is approximately 18 to 20 times smaller in area than the tympanic membrane, contributing significantly to the amplification of sound waves by the ear ossicles.

The middle ear ossicles are associated with two very small skeletal muscles (see Fig. 1–10). The tensor tympani muscle is a spherical muscle that attaches to the malleus by a short tendon. It is supplied by a branch of the trigeminal nerve. The stapedius, the smallest skeletal muscle in the body, is closely related to the facial nerve at its origin. This muscle is supplied by the facial nerve. Reflex contraction of these two muscles in response to loud noises results in fixation of the ear ossicles, damping vibrations. This protective reflex is called the *tympanic reflex*. It takes approximately 40 to 160 milliseconds for the tympanic reflex to occur.

Tympanic Bulla

The osteum of the auditory tube lies in a rostrodorsomedial location in the tympanic bulla, coursing anteriorly. The auditory tube is lined by pseudostratified ciliated columnar epithelium containing goblet cells. The auditory tube opens into the nasopharynx and equalizes air pressure on either side of the tympanic membrane. On the medial wall of the tympanic cavity is the promontory, a bony shelf that houses the bony labyrinth (see Fig. 1–10).

The central space of the labyrinth, called the *vestibule,* is continuous with the subarachnoid space via the cochlear aqueduct (see Fig. 1–10). It is filled with perilymph, which is similar to cerebrospinal fluid. The vestibule connects to the three semicircular canals and the cochlea.

On the lateral side of the promontory is a thin bony plate containing two windows or fenestrations. The oval or vestibular window lies on the dorsolateral surface of the promontory immediately adjacent to the pars flaccida. It attaches to the base of the stapes and connects to the vestibule. Vibrations are transmitted to the endolymph contained within the cochlea from the tympanic membrane via the ear ossicle chain to the oval window. The round window, an opening in the bony shelf of the osseous cochlea, is covered by a secondary tympanic membrane. It is found in the anterior end of the vestibule, just ventral to the smaller oval window. This membrane permits vibrations that have already passed to sensory receptors to be dissipated into the air-filled tympanic bulla.

The middle ear cavity of the cat is divided by a septum into two separate tympanic cavities (Fig. 1–12). In the small dorsolateral compartment lie the auditory ossicles, the osteum of the auditory tube, and the eardrum. The larger ventromedial compartment is an air-filled tympanic bulla. The two compartments of the tympanic bulla communicate via a small passage located dorsally near the cochlear window. This intervening bony septum should be perforated when necessary for proper drainage of the middle ear cavity. Rough handling of the bony septum may result in damage to the post-ganglionic sympathetic nerves. The nerves, which are visible submucosally as fine strands over the cochlear promontory, should be avoided during surgical removal of the septum in the cat.

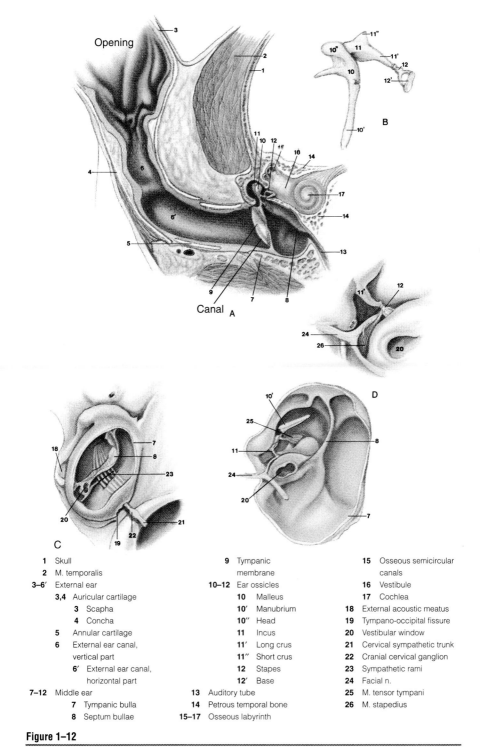

Opening

Canal A

B

D

C

1	Skull	**9**	Tympanic membrane	**15**	Osseous semicircular canals
2	M. temporalis			**16**	Vestibule
3–6'	External ear	**10–12**	Ear ossicles	**17**	Cochlea
3,4	Auricular cartilage	**10**	Malleus	**18**	External acoustic meatus
3	Scapha	**10'**	Manubrium	**19**	Tympano-occipital fissure
4	Concha	**10''**	Head	**20**	Vestibular window
5	Annular cartilage	**11**	Incus	**21**	Cervical sympathetic trunk
6	External ear canal, vertical part	**11'**	Long crus	**22**	Cranial cervical ganglion
6'	External ear canal, horizontal part	**11''**	Short crus	**23**	Sympathetic rami
		12	Stapes	**24**	Facial n.
7–12	Middle ear	**12'**	Base	**25**	M. tensor tympani
7	Tympanic bulla	**13**	Auditory tube	**26**	M. stapedius
8	Septum bullae	**14**	Petrous temporal bone		
		15–17	Osseous labyrinth		

Figure 1–12

Schematic views of cat middle and internal ear. (From Hudson LC, Hamilton WP: Atlas of Feline Anatomy for Veterinarians. Philadelphia, WB Saunders, 1993.)

Nerves

Two types of nerves should be considered in relation to the middle ear: (1) nerves in transit in close association with the middle ear but destined for a distant location and (2) nerves that play a role in normal function of the middle ear. All are susceptible to injury by disease of or trauma to the middle ear.

Those nerves that are in transit in relation to the middle ear are:

- The sympathetic post-ganglionic nerves to the eye and orbit from nerve cell bodies located in the cranial cervical ganglion
- The facial nerve and a branch from it (chorda tympani)
- A branch of the glossopharyngeal nerve

The sympathetic post-ganglionic nerve fibers are collectively called *internal carotid nerves* (see Fig. 1–11), and they travel as a perivascular nerve plexus along with internal carotid artery in the petro-occipital canal, which is separated from the middle ear cavity by a thin bony plate in the dog. Chronic infections in the middle ear cavity can erode the bone separating the carotid nerves from the middle ear cavity.

In the cat, the post-ganglionic sympathetic nerves run through the middle ear cavity submucosally below the septum of the tympanic bulla over the cochlear promontory. Damage to these nerves results in Horner's syndrome, consisting of miosis (constriction of the pupil) and enophthalmos (recession of the eyeball), contributing to prolapse of the third eyelid. Ptosis (drooping of the upper eyelid) may also be present.

The facial nerve travels through the bony facial canal (Fig. 1–13). As mentioned before, the facial canal is incomplete, exposing this nerve to the middle ear cavity. This can contribute to the involvement of the facial nerve in chronic middle ear infections. Early symptoms of facial nerve involvement may include blepharospasm. Other symptoms, such as drooping of the ear, paralysis of buccal muscles, and spasms of platysma behind the ear on the affected side, may also be exhibited, depending on the degree of facial nerve involvement.

The chorda tympani, a branch of the facial nerve, runs through the middle ear cavity. It courses medial to the base of the malleus in the dorsal compartment of the middle ear (see Figs. 1–10 and 1–13). The chorda tympani carries preganglionic parasympathetic nerves that synapse in the mandibular and sublingual ganglia to innervate the mandibular and sublingual salivary glands, respectively. This nerve also carries gustatory fibers from fungiform papillae in the rostral two thirds of the tongue. Because taste buds require neurotropic influences to remain functional, damage to the chorda tympani may result in atrophy of fungiform papillae on the affected side.

The tympanic nerve of the glossopharyngeal nerve supplies the mucous membrane lining of the tympanic bulla. The tympanic nerve gives off the tympanic plexus, which innervates the middle ear cavity (see Fig. 1–11).

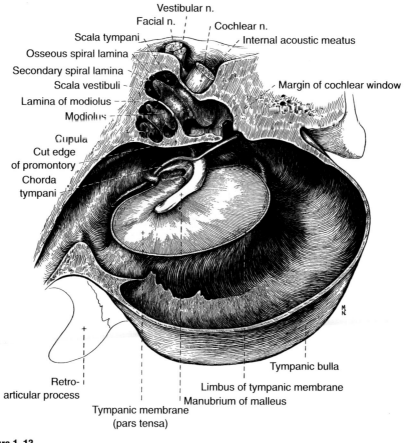

Vestibular n.
Facial n.
Cochlear n.
Scala tympani
Internal acoustic meatus
Osseous spiral lamina
Secondary spiral lamina
Scala vestibuli
Margin of cochlear window
Lamina of modiolus
Modiolus
Cupula
Cut edge
of promontory
Chorda
tympani
Tympanic bulla
Retro-
articular process
Limbus of tympanic membrane
Manubrium of malleus
Tympanic membrane
(pars tensa)

Figure 1–13

Sculpted medial view of the right middle ear and cochlea. (From Evans HE (ed): Miller's Anatomy of the Dog, 3rd ed. Philadelphia, WB Saunders, 1993.)

These nerves may be involved in sensing pressure changes across the tympanic membrane. They may also carry pain sensations from the middle ear cavity. The tympanic nerve itself runs through the middle ear cavity submucosally as the minor petrosal nerve, which mainly carries preganglionic parasympathetic nerve fibers to the otic ganglion. Post-ganglionic nerve fibers from the otic ganglion innervate the parotid and zygomatic salivary glands. Injury to the tympanic nerve may lead to partial loss of salivation on the affected side. The tensor *tympani* from the mandibular nerve of the trigeminal innervates the tensor tympani muscle. Stapedial nerves from the facial nerve provide motor innervation to the stapedius muscle. The tensor tympani and stapedial nerves are clinically not important.

Inner Ear

The main functions of the inner ear are receiving auditory signals and maintaining equilibrium. The inner ear is located within the osseous labyrinth of the petrous part of the temporal bone. The membranous labyrinth consists of three primary parts: the cochlea, vestibule, and semicircular canals. The vestibule is divided into an utricle and a saccule. The vestibulocochlear nerve (cranial nerve VIII) supplies the membranous cochlea, vestibule, and semicircular canals (Fig. 1–14).

Osseous Anatomy

The petrosal part of the tympanic bone has an internal pyramid containing the internal acoustic meatus, the osseous and membranous labyrinths, and an external mastoid process. The pyramidal part of the petrous (meaning "rocklike") temporal bone is the hardest bone in the body. The rostrodorsal surface of the pyramid is in contact with the cerebrum and hence is called the *cerebral surface,* whereas the caudomedial surface contacts the cerebellum and is called the *cerebellar surface.* The mid-part of the cerebellar surface of the pyramid exhibits a foramen called the *internal acoustic meatus.* The internal acoustic meatus in turn presents two tiny foramina: (1) a dorsally located foramen that leads into the osseous facial canal for the seventh cranial nerve and vestibular component of the eighth cranial nerve and (2) a ventrally located foramen for the cochlear component of the eighth cranial nerve (see Fig. 1–13). Because of the close association of the facial and eighth cranial nerves within the petrous temporal bone, the two nerves may be affected simultaneously by the same lesion.

The excavation within the petrous temporal bone, called the *osseous labyrinth,* is approximately 15 mm long. It is divided into three compartments: the cochlea, vestibule, and semicircular canals. The osseous vestibule is continuous with the subarachnoid space via the cochlear aqueduct (see Fig. 1–10). Via this duct, the perilymph is continuous with cerebrospinal fluid in the subarachnoid space surrounding the brain. Chronic middle ear infections can thus travel via the vestibular or

Figure 1–14

Schematic drawing of the inner ear. *Lower panel* shows innervation of the inner ear complex by branches of the eighth cranial nerve. The membranous labyrinth is rotated 180 degrees ventrodorsally. *Top panel* shows the membranous cochlea in section and the spiral organ (organ of Corti). *a,* tectorial membrane; *b,* vestibular membrane; *c,* spiral ganglion of cochlea; *d,* scala media; *e,* stria vascularis, which primarily produces endolymph; *f,* outer hair cells, which are sensory receptors for sound; *g,* basilar membrane.

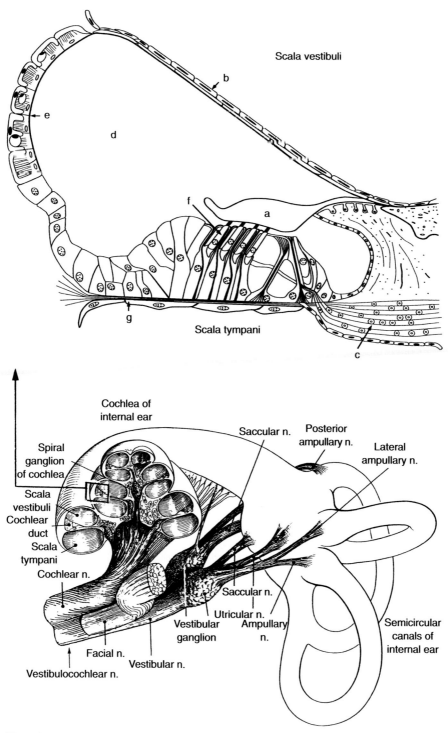

Scala vestibuli

b

e

d

f

a

g

Scala tympani

c

Cochlea of
internal ear

Saccular n.   Posterior
ampullary n.   Lateral
ampullary n.

Spiral
ganglion
of cochlea

Scala
vestibuli
Cochlear
duct
Scala
tympani

Cochlear n.

Saccular n.

Utricular n.
Vestibular   Ampullary
ganglion   n.

Semicircular
canals of
internal ear

Facial n.

Vestibular n.

Vestibulocochlear n.

Figure 1–14

See legend on opposite page

21

cochlear window to affect the inner ear and eventually can spread via the cochlear aqueduct to the meninges. Within the osseous labyrinth, the membranous labyrinth is suspended in perilymph.

Cochlea

The membranous labyrinth within the osseous labyrinth is an interconnecting system of epithelium-lined tubes and spaces filled with a clear fluid called *endolymph.* As mentioned before, the vestibule consists of the utricle and the saccule. These sacs communicate directly with each other and also with the semicircular and cochlear ducts. The cochlea is receptive to vibrations in endolymph, and the rest of the membranous labyrinth is associated with the function of equilibrium. Problems within the membranous labyrinth lead to signs of deafness and vestibular disease, including vestibular ataxia, circling, head tilting, strabismus, and nystagmus.

The bony cochlea winds around a hollow central axis *(modiolus)* in a dorsoventral direction. The modiolus accommodates the cochlear nerve (see Fig. 1–14). The *osseous* or *bony spiral lamina* is a bony shelf that projects from the modiolus into the interior of the canal. Like the cochlea, it makes three and a quarter turns to end at the apex (or *cupula;* see Fig. 1–13). The bony spiral lamina reaches about halfway into the lumen of the bony cochlea, partially dividing its cavity into two parts, the dorsal *scala vestibuli* and the ventral *scala tympani.*

The membranous cochlear duct is an epithelium-lined and endolymph-filled structure that extends from the osseous spiral lamina to the outer bony wall, completely dividing the scala vestibuli and scala tympani. The scala vestibuli and scala tympani are continuous with each other at the apex of the modiolus through a small foramen called the *helicotrema.* The cavity of the membranous cochlea, called the *scala media,* is filled by endolymph.

A specialized thickened epithelium in the basilar membrane constitutes the *spiral organ* (organ of Corti), in which cochlear nerve endings innervate the sensory hair cells. The hair cells are exposed to a specialized leaflike structure, the *tectorial membrane.* Vibrations of perilymph are transmitted to endolymph by the intervening (vestibular) membrane between the scala vestibuli and the scala media. The tectorial membrane in turn vibrates, touching the hair cells and initiating nerve impulses that are carried by the cochlear nerve to the brain.

Damage to the hair cells leads to hearing deficits or loss. Congenital deafness may be either perceptive (inner ear defect) or central (lesion of the auditory brain center). Acquired deafness may be either central or peripheral, resulting from chronic disease, normal aging, or drug use. Aminoglycoside therapy can lead to ototoxicity, a leading cause of iatrogenic hearing loss. White cats with congenital deafness have numerous cochlear abnormalities, including lesions in the spiral ganglion of the cochlear nerve.

References

Blauch B, Strafuss AC: Histologic relationships of the facial (7th) and vestibulocochlear (8th) cranial nerves within the petrous temporal bone in the dog. Am J Vet Res 35:481, 1974.

Evans HE: Miller's Anatomy of the Dog, 3rd ed. Philadelphia, WB Saunders, 1993.

Getty R: Sisson and Grossman's The Anatomy of the Domestic Animals, 5th ed, vol 2. Philadelphia, WB Saunders, 1975.

King AS, Riley VA: A Guide to the Physiological and Clinical Anatomy of the Head, 4th ed. Liverpool, University of Liverpool, 1980.

2

Examination of the External Ear Canal

Louis N. Gotthelf, DVM

O ne of the most common ailments of dogs seen in a veterinary practice is ear disease. Approximately 15% to 20% of all canine patients and approximately 6% to 7% of all feline patients have some kind of ear disease, from mild erythema to severe otitis media. Many clients are unaware of their pets' otitis, and many pets do not show clinical signs of ear disease until it has become quite severe. Determining the cause of ear disease is often a difficult task.

Examination of the ear canals and tympanic membranes of dogs and cats can be extremely frustrating for the veterinarian presented with a patient suffering from ear disease. Simply manipulating the pinna or inserting the otoscope cone into the painful ear of a dog or cat can cause discomfort to the patient and may result in aggressive behavior toward the examiner. Looking through an otoscope in a patient that is shaking its head to relieve its discomfort gives the examiner a very quick, superficial look, at best. Painful ears prevent thorough examination, so sedation or anesthesia is required for a complete examination.

The Normal Ear

To become familiar with the appearance of the normal ear canal and eardrum, the veterinarian should perform a thorough ear examination on every patient anesthetized for any reason (such as ovariohysterectomy or a dental procedure). Knowing (1) what the normal ear canal should look like, (2) where the eardrum should be located, if it is not readily visible, and (3) how to distinguish normal cerumen from otitic exudates is required to determine whether the ear is affected by disease.

Ear Canal

The normal ear canal epithelium should be light pink with small superficial blood vessels visible (Fig. 2–1). Small amounts of cerumen coating the epithelium give the surface a glistening appearance. Cerumen is a normal part of a healthy ear and should not be regarded as pathological unless it is excessive. Hairs are seen along the canal, being more numerous in the vertical canal (Fig. 2–2).

The dog's ear canal gently bends approximately 75 degrees as it changes from the vertical to the horizontal (Fig. 2–3). With the dog in the standing position, the examiner should gently place traction ventrally on the pinna; the ear canal will straighten out because the normal underlying cartilage is soft and pliable. The otoscope cone should be advanced into the horizontal canal as the canal straightens. This technique enables the horizontal canal to be examined. In the anesthetized patient in lateral recumbency, the examiner can straighten out the canal by lifting the pinna vertically to the point of elevating the entire head.

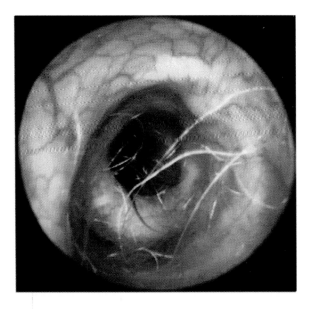

Figure 2–1

Normal ear canal of the dog.

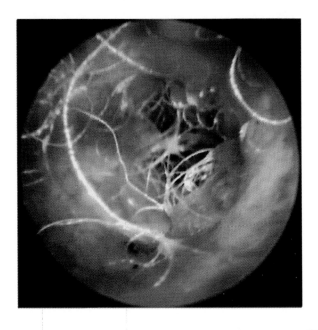

Figure 2–2

Numerous hairs and wax found in the vertical canal of a Poodle.

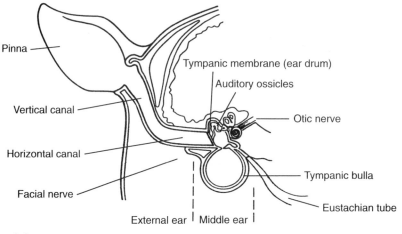

Pinna

Tympanic membrane (ear drum)

Auditory ossicles

Vertical canal

Otic nerve

Horizontal canal

Facial nerve

Tympanic bulla

Eustachian tube

External ear | Middle ear |

Figure 2–3

The anatomy of the ear canal. The vertical canal bends at approximately 75 degrees to become the horizontal canal.

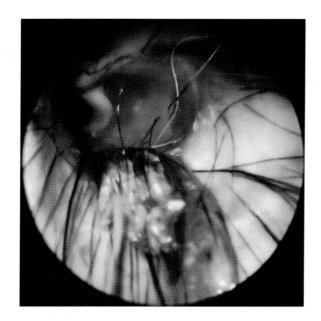

Figure 2–4

A tuft of long, thick, bristly hairs is sometimes found in the horizontal canal, originating near the annulus of the eardrum.

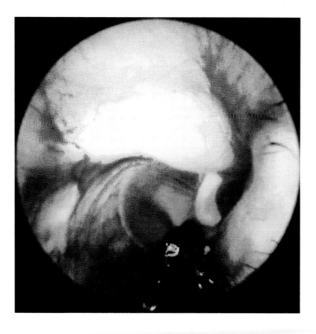

Figure 2–5

Accumulation of wax along the ventral floor of the horizontal canal. This wax is helpful for orienting the dorsoventral axis during examination of the ear canal.

Hairs are almost absent from the horizontal canal in most dogs. However, a clump of long, bristly hairs is often found at the distal end of the horizontal canal and may be causing discomfort (Fig. 2–4). An accumulation of wax may be seen along the ventral floor of the horizontal canal (Fig. 2–5). As the otoscope is advanced in the horizontal canal, the tympanic membrane, if present, should become visible.

Tympanic Membrane

The normal tympanic membrane in both the dog and the cat appears as a thin, transparent to translucent, reflective end of the horizontal ear canal (Figs. 2–6 and 2–7). The normal eardrum has been described as having a pale gray "rice paper" appearance. The outline of the footplate (manubrium) of the malleus is seen attached to the medial side of the tympanic membrane, frequently bulging outward (pars tensa). The malleus is seen as a thin rectangular white bone originating from the dorsal portion of the tympanic membrane and extending ventrally halfway across the membrane. The malleus is oriented dorsoventrally. The free distal end of the manubrium may have a gentle curve or a "hook"

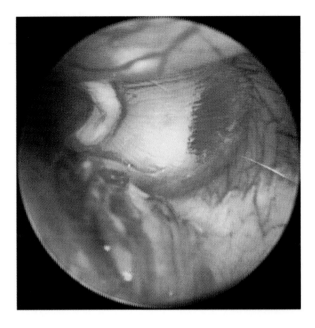

Figure 2–6

Normal canine eardrum. The yellow wax is in the ventral portion of the horizontal canal. The footplate of the malleus can be clearly seen through the rice paper–thin pars tensa. In the dorsal portion of the eardrum is the pars flaccida, with the blood vessels that supply the epithelium over the malleus.

that points rostrally. This feature aids in distinguishing the right ear from the left ear on photographs of the eardrum.

Examination of the dorsal portion of the tympanic membrane (pars flaccida) reveals an opaque, pink or white, loose membrane often containing a network of small blood vessels that extend across the tympanic membrane (Fig. 2–8). This "vascular strip" often has an edematous appearance and may obstruct visualization of dorsal portions of the eardrum. In many cases of otitis media, the vascular strip is destroyed, removing the blood supply to the germinal epithelium of the eardrum that is required for the eardrum to heal. If the vascular strip is unaffected by disease or trauma, the damaged eardrum has a much better chance of completely healing with time.

The tympanic membrane in some dogs is oriented at an acute angle of as much as 45 degrees to the long axis of the horizontal canal, making visualization of the entire eardrum difficult. Some dogs may have negative pressure in the tympanic bulla, which causes retraction of the eardrum into the bulla and makes examination difficult. A condition known as a "false middle ear" has been described, in which the tympanic membrane is actually stretched inward into the bulla and becomes attached to the

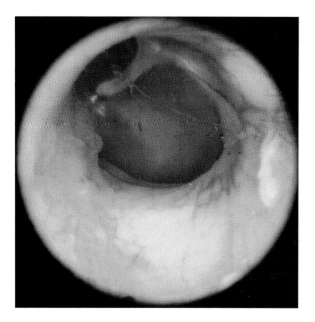

Figure 2–7

Normal feline eardrum.

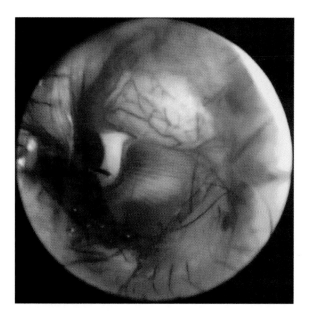

Figure 2–8

Prominent pars flaccida forming the "vascular strip." This provides the blood supply to the eardrum.

lining of the middle ear. In this condition, the entire middle ear cavity is obliterated. When such an ear is examined with the otoscope, no eardrum is seen, and a deep, dark hole is viewed.

In the anesthetized patient in lateral recumbency, the pinna is lifted vertically to straighten the curved ear canal, which makes advancing of the otoscope cone easier. The tip of the instrument can be advanced closer to the eardrum. The cat's tympanic membrane is easily visualized because the eardrum is oriented in a 90-degree plane with the ear canal.

Assessing the Ear Canals

With the otoscope, examiner evaluates the ear canals for:

- Patency or stenosis
- Color changes
- Proliferative changes
- Ulcerations
- Exudates (Fig. 2–9)
- Foreign bodies
- Parasites
- Tumors
- Excessive hair or waxy accumulation

Location of the lesion along the canal should be noted. If visibility is impaired by hair or excessive cerumen or exudate, then either plucking the hair plug or flushing the external ear canal is mandatory. Cytological and culture specimens of any exudate or secretions should be collected with a small cotton-tipped swab, curette, or catheter prior to initiation of any cleaning method.

In otitis externa, proteolytic enzymes are produced that have a depilatory effect, so hairs may be absent on examination. After therapy has resolved the ear disease, hair regrowth is a good indicator that the treatment was successful.

Flushing the Canals

Until a determination of the integrity of the eardrum is made, the choice of flushing solutions should be limited to nondetergent, non–alcohol-containing types of flushing solutions. Tepid solutions (98°F) of saline or very dilute povidone-iodine solution are used to soften and loosen wax and debris. Gentle flushing, using low pressure through either a Water Pik or a syringe and catheter, should be repeated until the ear canal is clean.

When ear disease is present, exudates accumulate along the ventral portion of the horizontal canal and remain in contact with the eardrum.

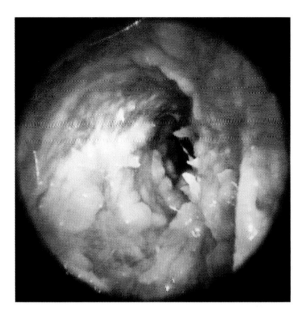

Figure 2–9

Otitis externa in a cocker spaniel. A yellow, creamy exudate is present in the vertical canal. This dog had a ceruminous otitis externa with large numbers of staphylococci.

Proteolytic enzymes elaborated as a result of inflammation break down the eardrum and weaken it. Therefore, even gentle flushing against a weakened membrane may cause it to rupture. Detergents and alcohols, along with many organic acids contained in ear cleaners, may gain access to the middle ear in this manner and are extremely irritating to the mucosa lining the bulla. If this should happen, the tympanic bulla should be copiously irrigated with normal saline.

If the eardrum is visible and is normal, detergent and alcohol-containing types of ear cleaners are safe to use for flushing of the ear canals. Ear curettes of various sizes can be used to scrape large pieces of exudate off the ear canal.

The Video Otoscope

A videographic otoscope (MedRx Video Vetscope, MedRx, Inc., Seminole, FL) is a very useful instrument for cleaning, drying, and examining the ear canal because it gives the examiner a clear real-time image on a video monitor (Fig. 2–10). The high-quality glass lens pack configured within the Video Vetscope probe begins with a 2-mm lens at the tip of the 4.75-mm diameter probe. This lens configuration provides a 60-degree angle of view and provides an in-focus image 2 to 3 inches ahead of the

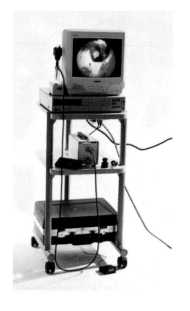

Figure 2-10

The Video Vetscope (a videographic otoscope), manufactured by MedRx, Inc., Seminole, FL.

probe tip. Even in small patients in which the ear canal diameter is smaller than the tip of the probe, the wide viewing angle of this instrument allows examination of the ear canal. Light fibers, connected to a 150-watt light source, are also at the tip of the probe and provide superior illumination. The entire instrument is attached to a miniature color video camera (Fig. 2–11), which is connected to a video monitor and a video printer.

For suctioning of the ear canals, the video otoscope has a 2-mm working channel through which a 5.5-inch, open-ended tomcat catheter or a 3F

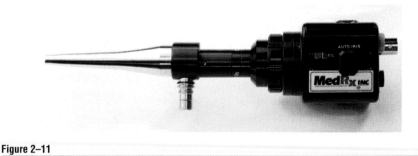

Figure 2-11

Video Vetscope and miniature video camera.

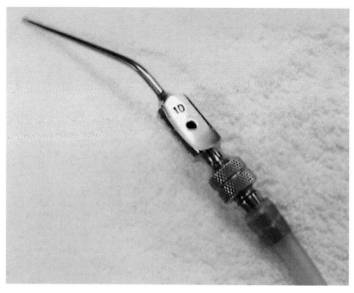

Figure 2–12

Number 10 Frazier suction tip connected to a suction machine. The free end connects to the flared end of the tomcat catheter.

feeding or urethral tube can be inserted. A No. 10 Frazier suction-tip catheter is used to connect the tubing from the suction machine to the catheter (Fig. 2–12). The catheter is inserted into the working channel with the otoscope positioned in the ear canal. The catheter can be advanced into the ear canal with clear visualization (Fig. 2–13). Small pieces of epithelium, wax, hairs, and pus can be suctioned out of the canal while the examiner views the procedure on the video monitor. In this manner, even the smallest pieces of detritus can be removed. The examiner can extract large pieces of debris and concretions of wax and medications from the ear canal under visualization with this instrument by using a grasping type of endoscopic forceps inserted through the 2-mm working channel (Fig. 2–14).

The video otoscope also has documentation capability. When a lesion is encountered, the image on the video monitor can be "frozen" and then printed out as a 4 × 5-inch color glossy photograph with the use of a video printer. Thus, there is a photographic hard copy document of the ear disease to place in the medical record for comparison on rechecks. These photographs are also helpful in counseling owners and showing them the severity of the ear disease; they also make the veterinarian's medical or surgical recommendations more valid. Documentation capability is very useful in a referral practice. The referring veterinarian can receive a color

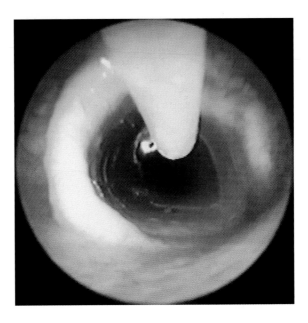

Figure 2-13

The open-ended tomcat catheter is advanced through the 2-mm channel of the Video Vetscope toward the flush solution. Advancing the catheter allows visualization of the suctioning process. (MedRx, Inc., Seminole, FL.)

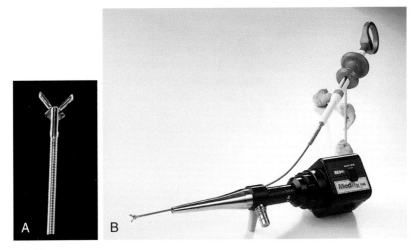

Figure 2-14

An oval fenestrated endoscopic grasping forceps (A) can be threaded through the Video Vetscope (B) for removal of foreign bodies, wax, polyps, and other material in the ear canal. (MedRx, Inc., Seminole, FL.)

photograph of the ear canal in addition to the written report. The photographs can also be used to illustrate contributions to veterinary medical literature. The video otoscope can also be coupled to a videorecorder so that the examination and surgical procedures can be videotaped and kept for documentation.

After the ear canal is cleaned and examined, the examiner can gain a better understanding of the ear disease and can better formulate therapeutic protocols.

Assessing the Eardrum

In most cases of chronic canine otitis media, the eardrum is ruptured as a result of long-standing otitis externa. Examination of the ears of a patient with chronic otitis media often reveals the absence of the eardrum. The tympanic bulla may be filled with a dark material composed of epithelial cells, keratin, and cerumen (Fig. 2–15). In acute otitis media, copious exudate resembling curdled milk is seen along the floor of the horizontal canal. Flecks of material are often seen floating in the liquid. After exudate and flush solution are suctioned from the external

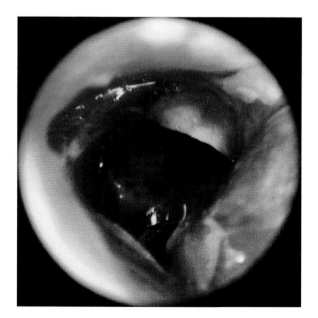

Figure 2–15

Appearance of the ear in otitis media. Otoscopic examination in a Toy Poodle revealed the absence of most of the eardrum. The pars flaccida can be seen in the dorsal portion of the annulus. The tympanic bulla is filled with a dark, waxy material composed of squamous epithelium, keratin, and cerumen.

ear canal, the eardrum may not be visualized, but the bony tympanic bulla can be visualized beyond the annulus of the tympanic membrane.

It is difficult to assess the integrity of the eardrum if this structure cannot be clearly seen. When stenosis or occlusion of the ear canal prevents visualization of the eardrum, a rigid tomcat catheter can be advanced through the stenosis carefully. As the catheter is slowly advanced, it encounters a hard object. If pressure is applied, there is resistance, and then the catheter advances; the eardrum was intact and the catheter has just perforated it. If the catheter hits a hard object and does not advance, the object usually is the medial wall of the tympanic bulla, and the eardrum is not intact.

Alternatively, if there is a small hole in the eardrum, the ear canal can be filled with normal saline with the patient in lateral recumbency and the affected ear facing upward. The video otoscope is advanced through the saline toward the eardrum. Any rising air bubbles indicate that air from within the tympanic cavity is escaping through a hole in the tympanic membrane.

Pathological changes may be present in the bulla and eardrum as indicated by opacity or discoloration of the intact eardrum (Fig. 2–16). These findings signify either an ascending otitis media, which is rare in the dog, or an otitis media in which the eardrum has healed over, leaving material

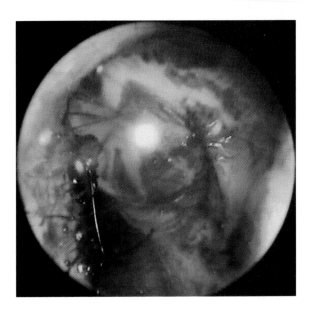

Figure 2–16

Change in shape and color of the eardrum. Bulging eardrum in a 6-month-old golden retriever with purulent exudate behind the eardrum.

within the tympanic bulla. The eardrum may be reddened in response to inflammation or from accumulation of blood in the bulla. Whitish opacity indicates pus or mucus in the bulla, and yellow a serous effusion. A bulging membrane signifies fluid pressure behind the eardrum. Retraction of the eardrum around the malleus indicates negative air pressure from eustachitis. To relieve pressure gradients and to obtain specimens from the middle ear for cytological evaluation and culture, a myringotomy should be done.

Myringotomy

Myringotomy is performed at the 5 o'clock or 7 o'clock position in the ventral portion of the pars tensa at the ventral-most portion of the attachment of the eardrum to the annulus (Fig. 2–17). Using this location for myringotomy prevents compromise of the blood supply to the eardrum and does not disrupt sound transmission from the malleus to the cochlea. The end of a 5.5-inch rigid, open-ended tomcat catheter is cut at a 45-degree angle so that there is a point at the tip. Long, thin (22-gauge) spinal needles are more expensive but may also be used for myringotomy.

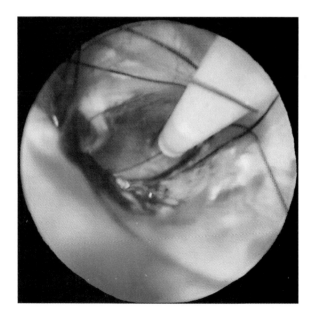

Figure 2–17

Using the open-ended tomcat catheter to perform a myringotomy. The catheter is positioned under visualization at the 5 o'clock position. A gentle push on the catheter makes a small perforation in the eardrum. The malleus and vascular strip are visible to the left of the catheter in the dorsum of the eardrum.

The pointed tip is then directed to the puncture site and is pushed through the eardrum to obtain specimens from the middle ear for cytological evaluation and culture. Irrigation and suction of the bulla can be performed from the same perforation site, and topical medications can be infused directly into the bulla. In most dogs, small myringotomy incisions completely heal within a month.

A small Buck curette can also be used to make a hole in the eardrum. This instrument makes a larger hole in the eardrum and is more difficult to accurately direct to the proper site for puncture. This technique may be used to create a large hole in the eardrum to allow middle ear exudates to drain into the horizontal canal and to prevent pressure gradients from recurring. Larger instruments and cotton-tipped swabs should not be used for myringotomy because they may tear the eardrum.

Cytological Evaluation

Cytological examination of specimens from every infected ear should be routine. Information gained from studying the cellular components of ear exudates becomes an integral part of the decision-making process in the treatment of ear disease.

Cytological specimens are obtained from the proximal horizontal canal and prepared as follows:

1. A small cotton-tipped swab is inserted into the ear without touching the ear canal. A plastic otoscope speculum is helpful to shroud the ear swab.

2. The sample is obtained by pressing the applicator tip against the ear canal as the swab is withdrawn. With this approach, packing of wax and exudate is minimal.

3. The swab is rolled onto a clean microscope slide; the harvested material from the left ear is rolled onto the left side of the slide, and the material from the right ear onto the right side of the slide.

4. The slide is labeled with the patient's name and the date of the sample (Fig. 2–18).

5. The slide is heat-fixed and stained with a blood stain (Diff-Quik or Wright-Giemsa stain).

6. After the slide is dried, a drop of slide-mounting medium (Cytoseal 60, Stephens Scientific, Riverdale, NJ) is applied, and a coverslip is placed over the material.

In this manner, a permanent slide is made. A drop of mineral oil can be spread on the slide if permanent slides are not desired. This standardized approach to making slides allows uniform identification of organisms from each ear and allows comparison of cytological findings from visit to visit.

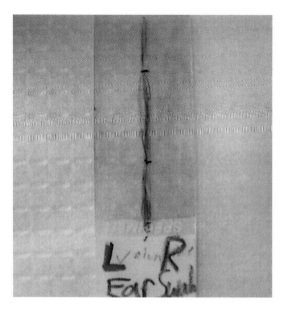

Figure 2–18

Roll-smear cytological slide. The left ear canal and right ear canal are labeled on the microscope slide as a means of standardizing cytological examination of each ear.

Evaluation of slides should begin with a low-power (100×) overview of the cell types. If there are large numbers of epithelial cells and few microorganisms, noninfectious causes of otitis such as seborrheic conditions should be considered (Fig. 2–19). High-power (400×) examination is needed to characterize bacteria and yeasts. Large numbers of bacteria or yeasts represent secondary invaders (Fig. 2–20). When neutrophils are seen in addition to bacteria or yeasts, infection and inflammation of subcutaneous tissues must be considered (Fig. 2–21). Ear mites are not often seen on stained ear swabs, but the eggs may be found. Clumps and clusters of epithelial cells may indicate neoplasia. Inflammatory cells and acantholytic cells may signify autoimmune disease.

To look for ear mites under the microscope, the examiner rolls swabs onto a slide containing a drop of mineral oil and applies a coverslip. Low-power examination reveals mites scurrying around on the slide, along with typical long oval eggs in the field (Fig. 2–22).

Skin Diseases Affecting the Ear

Pets with itchy ears may not have ear disease at all but may be responding to a localized pruritus associated with an underlying pruritic skin

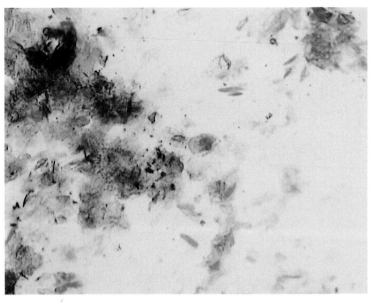

Figure 2–19

Low-power (100×) view of a roll smear. The predominant cell type is an unstained epithelial cell. This type of cytological presentation represents desquamated epithelial cells and sebaceous epithelial secretion.

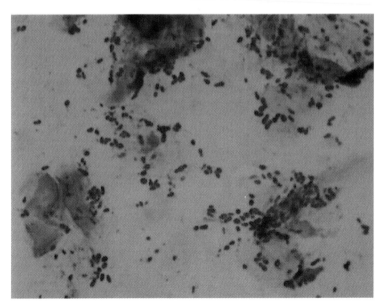

Figure 2–20

Large numbers of *Malassezia* yeasts are seen on this roll-smear cytological slide. Yeast organisms can be seen colonizing epithelial cells and free in the background.

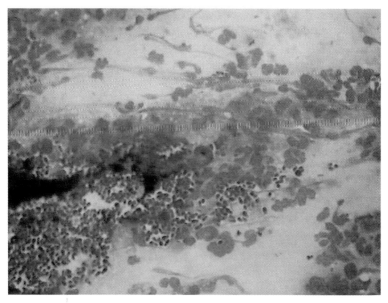

Figure 2–21

Neutrophils are seen on this slide along with large numbers of budding *Malassezia* yeasts from a patient with deep-seated otitis externa.

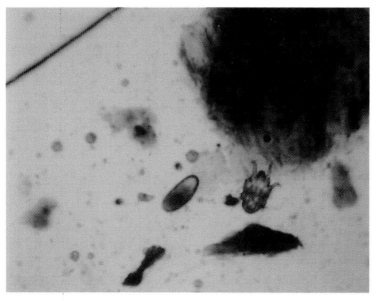

Figure 2–22

Ear mite *(Otodectes cyanotis)* and mite egg on mineral oil preparation from a cat with ear mites.

disease. Because many diseases found in the ear arise as a result of an underlying skin disease, the veterinarian should also carefully evaluate the pet's skin to determine the underlying cause if possible. Often, treatment for atopy, food allergy, or hypothyroidism diminishes the severity of the ear disease.

Suggested Readings

August JR: Evaluation of the Patient with Otitis Externa. Dermatology Reports, Solvay Veterinary, Vol 5, No 2, 1986.

Kwochka KW: Mites and related disease. Vet Clin North Am Small Anim Pract 17:1263–1284, 1987.

Little CJL, Lane JG: An evaluation of tympanometry, otoscopy, and palpation for assessment of the canine tympanic membrane. Vet Rec 124:5–8, 1989.

Reedy LM, Miller WH: Allergic Skin Diseases of Dogs and Cats. Philadelphia, WB Saunders, 1989, p 189.

Simpson D: Atresia of the external acoustic meatus in a dog. Austr Vet J 75:18–20, 1997.

Sirigu P, Perra MT, Ferelli C: Local immune response in the skin of the external auditory meatus: An immunohistochemical study. Microsc Res Tech 38:329–334, 1997.

Stout-Graham M, Kainer RA, Whalen LR, Macy DW: Morphologic measurements of the external horizontal ear canal of dogs. Am J Vet Res 51:990–994, 1990.

3

Factors That Predispose the Ear to Otitis Externa

Louis N. Gotthelf, DVM

Careful examination of a clean, dry ear canal in a dog or cat with otitis externa may reveal many conditions that affect the ear canal. Because the ear canal lining is actually modified skin, the same basic types of lesions found on the skin of the trunk may be found in the ear canal. Certain conditions, called *predisposing factors,* are responsible for altering the anatomy and physiology of the ear canal and increasing the likelihood of otitis externa.

For example, excessive skin folds at the base of the tail may predispose the English bulldog to a tail fold pyoderma. In the ear of this breed, excessive skin folds also predispose to otitis. The presence of a predisposing factor in a patient makes the ears more susceptible to otitis externa even when the patient is not exhibiting symptoms of otitis externa. By analogy, not all English bulldogs with excessive tail folds suffer from tail fold pyoderma. Because such dogs have the predisposing factor (the excessive folds), tail fold pyoderma is more likely to occur in this breed than in the beagle, which has no tail folds.

The floppy ear carriage common to many dog breeds predisposes the pet to otitis because of inadequate ventilation of the ear canal, which ultimately leads to higher humidity there. The dark, warm, moist area increases the chance that bacteria and yeasts will have a more favorable environment for growth and reproduction. It is not surprising that the incidence and severity of otitis externa are greater in dog breeds with floppy ears. Many of the floppy-eared breeds also have the predisposing factor of excessive hair growth in their ears. Cats and many dog breeds have erect ears that are well ventilated, and these pets have a lower incidence of otitis externa.

In developing a therapeutic plan for otitis externa, the veterinarian must give attention to the treatment of predisposing factors to effectively reduce the likelihood that the patient's ear disease will become chronic or recurrent. Some treatments to remove predisposing factors are very simple, such as plucking the excessive hairs found in a poodle's ears to reduce the humidity within the ear canal. Some breeders and veterinarians advocate taping or fixation of the ears of a Cocker spaniel over the top of its head to allow ear canal ventilation. Treatment of other predisposing factors is not such a simple matter. Diffuse cerumen gland adenocarcinoma, for example, requires total ear canal ablation to resolve.

Among the conditions found in the ear canals of dogs and cats that are considered to be predisposing factors favoring the development of otitis externa are:

- Stenosis
- Excessive hair
- Excessive cerumen production
- Any trauma to the ear canal
- Obstruction by tumor, polyp, or excessive granulation tissue

These anatomical and physiological alterations create a favorable climate for the proliferation of infectious organisms. High temperature and humidity in the ear canal, greater amounts of substrates for growth of bacteria and yeasts, and damaged epithelium result in the failure of the ear's normal immune mechanisms. Commensal bacteria and yeasts may be induced to reproduce in the favorable climate created. Otitis externa is the eventual result.

How does the presence of a predisposing factor in a patient's ear canal affect the course of otitis externa? Some pathophysiological mechanisms have been explained, but other mechanisms still remain a challenge. An understanding of the mechanisms involved in how these predisposing factors affect the normal physiology of the ear canal helps clinicians formulate more complete therapeutic plans for the treatment of otitis externa.

The normally smooth epithelial surface of the ear canal has a mechanism for clearing surface debris out of the ear canal; the process has been termed *epithelial migration*. Surface keratinocytes slowly slide along the epidermal layer of the ear canal, carrying cerumen and microorganisms out of the ear canal. When the anatomy of the epithelium of the ear canal

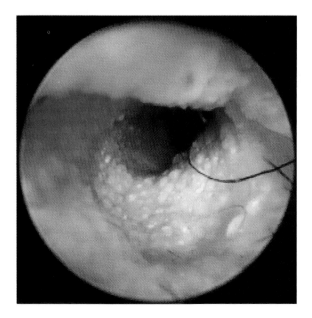

Figure 3–1

Otitis externa in a 6-month-old Yorkshire terrier. The ear canal epithelium is roughened in response to *Malassezia* otitis externa. Elevations and depressions are easily seen. Epithelial migration stops in these recesses. Bacteria and yeasts accumulate in the depressions and predispose this ear to otitis.

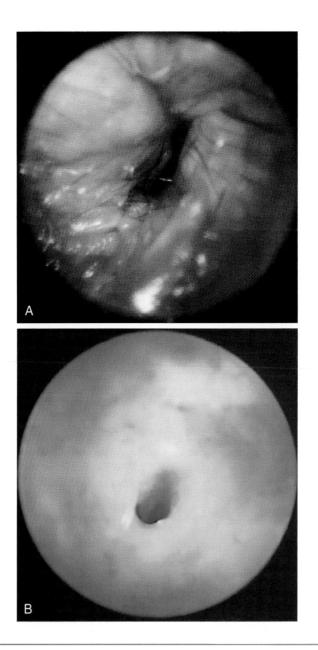

Figure 3–2

A, Stenosis of the vertical canal due to edema in a Cocker spaniel. *B,* Stenosis of the horizontal canal of a poodle as a result of subcutaneous chronic granulation tissue formation and replacement of the epithelial layer by fibrosis.

is altered by the presence of abnormal tissue, the movement of keratinocytes is also altered. The smooth surface of the normal ear canal becomes roughened or obstructed, and the debris accumulates at the point where the epithelial movement stops (Fig. 3–1). Inflammation and colonization of microorganisms occur at these points.

Stenotic Ear Canals

A common finding in dogs with otitis externa is a narrowed ear canal. Within the tube of skin that makes up the external ear canal, any swelling translates to decreasing lumen diameter. When the lumen of the ear canal becomes narrowed or occluded, stenosis results (Fig. 3–2). The stenosis magnifies the severity of the ear disease, making examination and treatment of the otitis externa more difficult.

A brief review of the anatomy of the external ear canal is helpful in delineating the mechanisms involved in creating the stenotic ear canal. The ear canal of the dog is lined by keratinizing stratified squamous epithelium.

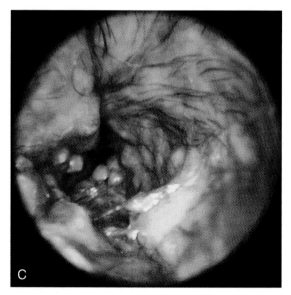

Figure 3–2 *Continued*

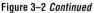

C, Stenosis at the junction of the vertical and horizontal ear canals of a mixed-breed dog as a result of small cerumen gland adenomas occluding the lumen of the ear canal.

Vertical Ear Canal

The skin of the vertical canal is approximately 1 mm thick and contains a well-developed dermis and subcutaneous layer. Numerous long, coarse hairs are present along the vertical canal. Surrounding the hair follicles are numerous sebaceous and ceruminous glands (modified apocrine glands). No eccrine sweat glands are located in the external ear canal. Hairs are most numerous toward the opening of the ear canal, and the number of hairs decreases along the ear canal toward the eardrum. Conversely, the ceruminous glands increase in density in the vertical canal distally.

The external acoustic meatus and the skin on the pinna contain numerous adnexal structures and have a significant subcutaneous layer, which can respond to disease. Frequently, the stenotic portion of the ear is limited only to the external acoustic meatus (Fig. 3–3). In that situation, the otoscope tip may be passed through the stenosis, revealing a normal vertical canal beyond it.

The ear canal of the Shar Pei has an abundant mucinous dermis under the epithelial layer that increases the thickness and folding of the

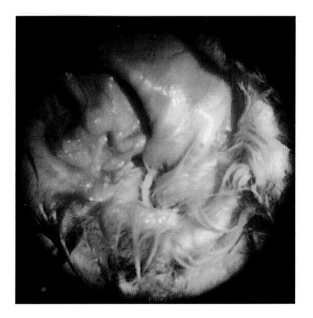

Figure 3–3

Stenosis of the external acoustic meatus. Inflammation and edema of the skin surround the entrance to the ear canal in an Old English sheepdog with acute moist dermatitis ("hot spot") on the lateral aspect of the face.

dermal-epidermal layer. Owing to the anatomically normal thick lining, the lumen diameter in this breed is decreased. The Shar Pei's ear canal is thus predisposed to higher humidity and greater glandular secretions, promoting bacterial and yeast colonization.

Anatomically, the vertical canal is more prone to becoming stenotic because of the vascularity and glandular structures found there. The inflammation and edema lead to narrowing of the ear canal. The stenosis prevents drainage of exudates out of the ear canal and complicates therapy by preventing topical medications from achieving therapeutic levels beyond the stenotic portion. Increases in fluid and air pressure beyond the stenosis can cause excessive pressure on the eardrum, predisposing it to rupture.

Inflammation and edema increase the thickness of the subcutaneous layer of the ear canal leading to stenosis. Chronic otitis externa leads to progressive pathological changes of the lining epithelium such as hyperkeratosis and hyperplasia (Fig. 3–4). The marked thickening of the epithelial layer may significantly reduce ear canal diameter. Increases in the number and size of sebaceous glands (Fig. 3–5) and dilated apocrine glands also reduce lumen diameter (Fig. 3–6). In addition, pathological changes that lead to calcification (Fig. 3–7) and thickening of the auricu-

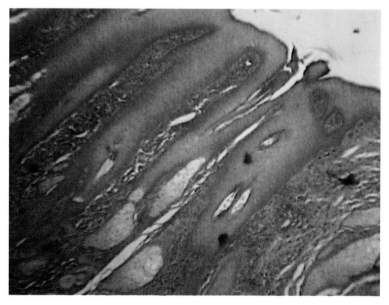

Figure 3–4

Photomicrograph of a biopsy specimen of a stenotic ear canal with epithelial hyperplasia due to chronic otitis externa. There are deep rete ridges and numerous layers to the epithelium. Inflammatory cells have infiltrated the dermis. Note the small sebaceous glands.

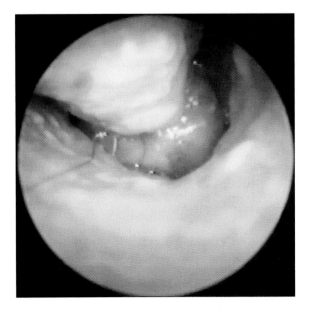

Figure 3–5

Stenosis of the vertical ear canal of a Shetland sheepdog. Otoscopic examination revealed obliteration of the ear canal lumen by increased tissue thickness. No infection was present in this ear. Total ear canal ablation was performed to give relief to this patient.

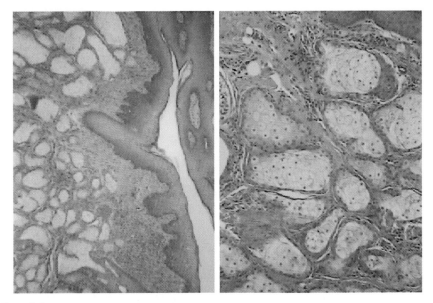

Figure 3–6

Histopathological section from the Shetland sheepdog ear canal shown in Figure 3–5. There is a mild epithelial hyperplasia *(left side)* and small lumen diameter. A substantial increase in the number and size of the sebaceous glands is present in the subcutaneous tissue *(right side)*. This is a case of sebaceous gland hyperplasia.

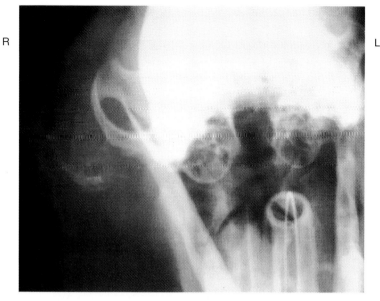

R   L

Figure 3-7

Open-mouth radiographic view of the thickened right tympanic bulla and calcified ear canal in a Cocker spaniel that was presented with a stenotic ear canal of the right ear. The dog had a great deal of pain. Medical therapy for 2 years had proved unsuccessful. Vertical ear canal ablation was performed to remove the calcified aural tissue. At surgery, the horizontal ear canal was found to be spared of stenosis or inflammation. A plug of desquamated epithelial tissue was found residing in the horizontal canal, and the eardrum was ruptured.

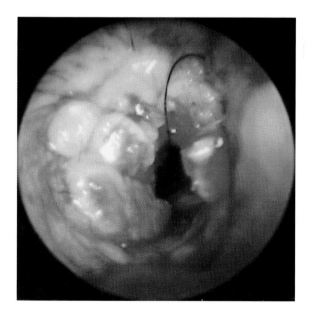

Figure 3-8

Chronic, ulcerating granulation tissue caused stenosis of the horizontal ear canal in a mixed-breed dog.

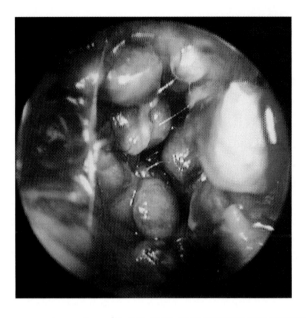

Figure 3–9

Cerumen gland adenomas in a Cocker spaniel. Large, multiple tumors are present in the vertical ear canal, causing a stenotic ear canal. This dog had chronic bacterial otitis, which was continuously treated with twice-weekly ear flushes and topical antibiotics. The owner declined surgery.

lar cartilage (especially in Cocker spaniels) or to fibrosis and formation of excessive granulation tissue resulting from chronic infection also lead to narrowing of the ear canal lumen (Fig. 3–8). Tumors such as ceruminous adenocarcinoma may also occlude the ear canal lumen (Fig. 3–9).

Horizontal Ear Canal

Fortunately, the skin of the horizontal canal is often spared the devastating effects of inflammation associated with otitis externa. The thin epidermis lining the horizontal canal firmly attaches to the underlying auricular cartilage in the lateral aspect of the horizontal canal (cartilaginous portion) and is approximately 0.2 mm thick. The medial portion of the horizontal canal has an extension of the petrous temporal bone underlying the thin epidermis (bony portion). The thin epithelium of the bony horizontal canal is continuous with the epithelium on the lateral aspect of the tympanic membrane, which is one or two cells thick. Epidermal rete ridges, skin adnexal structures, and a subcutaneous layer are absent in the skin of the horizontal canal. Because the skin is adherent to the underlying cartilage and to the periosteum of the bony portion of the horizontal canal, pathological changes of the horizontal canal are usually limited to hyperplasia.

Overtreatment

Long-standing overtreatment of ears with ear cleaners may macerate the epithelium, causing swelling and greater folding of the epithelial surface. Drugs such as neomycin are known to trigger a contact dermatitis within the ear canal, leading to erythema and swelling in the ear canal. If either of these causes is suspected, suspending all topical treatment for 1 to 2 weeks may decrease the tissue reaction and relieve the stenosis.

Stenosis

Stenosis presents a special problem in examination of the ear canal. Instruments cannot be inserted through the narrowed canal, and the integrity of the eardrum cannot be determined otoscopically. Occasionally, a short course of potent corticosteroids, applied topically, injected directly into the stenotic tissue, or administered parenterally, decreases the inflammatory infiltrates and reduces edema (Fig. 3–10). In addition, corticosteroids decrease the amounts of glandular secretions, make them less viscous so that they are easier to flush out of the ear canal, and reduce the secretion and dilation of ceruminous glands. If corticosteroids successfully increase the lumen diameter, adequate visualization of the ear canal and tympanic membrane becomes possible.

When medical therapy for stenosis is ineffective because of severe pathological changes to the ear canal, surgical ablation of the vertical canal, horizontal canal, or both is required. Surgical treatment of stenotic ears relieves the pain associated with chronic otitis and allows the remaining ear canal to be ventilated.

Hair in Ear Canals

In some of the haired breeds, such as the poodle and many of the terriers, long hairs normally grow from the skin of the ear canal. The number of hair follicles in predisposed breeds gradually decreases along the length of the external ear canal. The highest density of hair follicles occurs at the entrance to the ear canals at the pinna and along the proximal portion of the vertical canal. Occasional hairs may be found along the deeper parts of the canal.

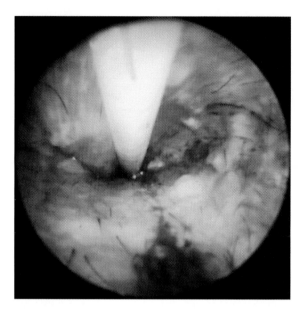

Figure 3–10

Infusion of corticosteroids beyond a stenotic portion of the ear canal. A tomcat catheter (5F) is placed through the stenosis until resistance is met. A potent corticosteroid solution (dexamethasone, betamethasone, fluocinolone) in a syringe attached to the catheter is infused through the catheter until it flushes back from the stenosis. Such infusions are often effective in reducing inflammation and edema to allow otoscopic examination.

Excessive hair or knots of ear hair may occlude the ear canals and interfere with adequate drying of the canal. The excessive moisture created by hair plugs predisposes these breeds to otitis externa. Certain bacteria, such as *Pseudomonas* and *Proteus,* thrive in a humid ear canal. When long hairs become matted and tangled in the ear canal, cerumen, exudates, and other secretions mold to the hair mass and form an occlusion.

Routine plucking of hairs by groomers may not be necessary in a dog whose ears are normal, and can sometimes be detrimental. In a dog that has recurrent ear infections and excessive hair growth in the ear canal, however, the hair should be routinely removed to prevent a mass of tangled hairs from blocking the ear canal lumen. Plucking the excessive hairs from the ears in breeds predisposed to otitis externa is recommended for the prevention and management of otitis externa.

Excessive Cerumen Production

The external ear canal is lined with both sebaceous and apocrine glands. The sebaceous glands are relatively superficial, surround hair follicles, and have ducts that open into the hair follicle below the surface of the epithelium. The apocrine (tubular) glands are located in the deeper dermis, are unassociated with hair follicles, and are often referred to as the *ceruminous glands* (Fig. 3–11).

Cerumen is primarily a lipid-containing material produced by the secretory products of both of these types of glands. The sebaceous gland is a holocrine gland. Its secretion is composed of disintegrating desquamated glandular epithelial cells. The apocrine glandular secretion is a waxy acellular liquid. Cerumen, then, is composed of a mixture of sebaceous epithelial cells suspended in apocrine lipid secretion. Imbalances in the ratio of the secretions of these two types of glands may play a role in otitis externa.

As the number of hairs decreases along the length of the vertical ear canal, the number of sebaceous glands also decreases. The ceruminous glands are numerous along both the haired and nonhaired portions of the vertical ear canal.

Some authorities suggest that there are actually two types of cerumen, liquid and dry. In humans, it is thought that residents of Arctic climates favor the dry cerumen, whereas those who reside in temperate or equatorial climates tend to have the more liquid cerumen. The author has ob-

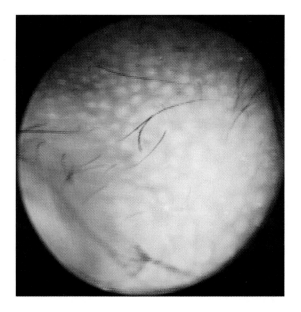

Figure 3–11

Dilated apocrine tubular glands are numerous in the ear of a 5-month-old Cocker spaniel with ceruminous otitis externa. The ceruminous glands are unassociated with hair follicles. Only a few hairs are present, but there is a large number of dilated glands.

served both dry and wet cerumen in dogs and cats (Figs. 3–12 and 3–13). Whether this is a genetic predisposition, as suggested in humans, or a feature of certain ear diseases has not been determined.

The hydrophobic properties of normal cerumen make it an important barrier to the entry of excessive moisture to the epithelial cells of the external ear canal. Certain components of normal cerumen, such as lysozyme and interleukins, are thought to provide an antibacterial and antiviral characteristic to cerumen. Routine ear cleaning in normal dogs and cats, which removes these important immunologic factors, is not necessary and may even predispose to otitis externa.

Under normal circumstances, cerumen that is produced along the vertical canal is transported laterally along the canal wall toward the pinna in conjunction with normal epithelial migration and is subsequently extruded. If cotton-tipped applicators are used to clean an ear canal full of cerumen and other debris, the material can be pushed toward the horizontal canal and eardrum, resulting in cerumen impaction. This condition is best treated with ceruminolytic agents or curettage of the inspissated cerumen.

A condition known as *failure of epithelial migration* results when the normal cerumen clearance mechanism is disrupted. Normally, keratinocytes originating from the central portion of the eardrum slide along

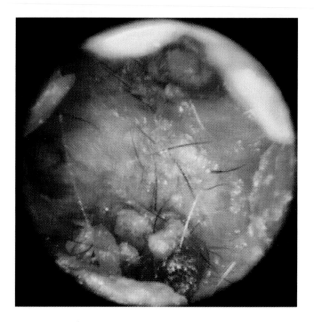

Figure 3–12

Dry, flaky cerumen in sheets and small clumps.

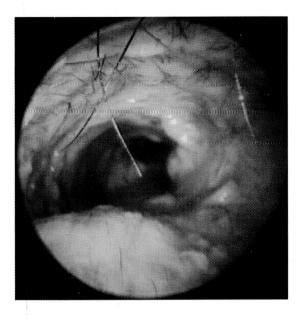

Figure 3–13

Wet cerumen. The uniform coating of cerumen in this ear canal gives it a glistening, moist appearance.

the basal epithelium in the superficial layers along the entire ear canal and carry cerumen from the eardrum to the pinna. Damage to the eardrum prevents the migration of these cells, allowing layering rather than promoting clearing of cerumen. The resulting accumulation can become quite large (Fig. 3–14). Such *ceruminoliths* may be removed from the surface of the eardrum with a grasping forceps. Occasionally, soft cerumen makes grasping the entire cerumen plug impossible. These plugs are best prepared for removal by using warm flushing solution to soften the wax. Curettes and large-bore catheters connected to suction aid in their removal.

Certain breeds predisposed to otitis externa, such as the Cocker spaniel, Springer spaniel, and Labrador retriever, have a higher number of apocrine glands in the dermis of their ear canals than other breeds. A greater area of apocrine glands may be a predisposing factor in otitis externa. The density of glandular tissue is significantly higher in the vertical (proximal) ear canal, with a scarcity of glandular tissue and hair follicles in the horizontal (distal) ear canal. In the presence of otitis externa, however, the distal ear canal may also become infiltrated by distended apocrine glands. Cystic ceruminous glands called *apocrine cysts* are sometimes found in the ear canal (Fig. 3–15).

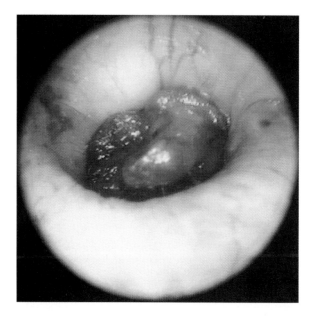

Figure 3–14

Cerumen accumulation at the eardrum of a dog. The ear canal seems unaffected by any type of disease. It is thought that the wax accumulates on a damaged portion of the eardrum.

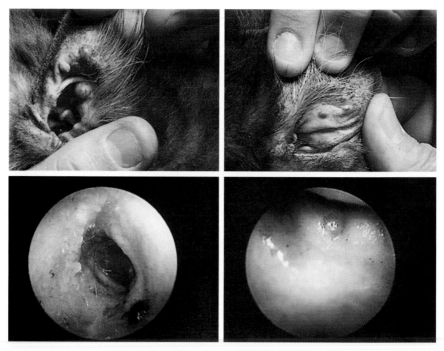

Figure 3–15

Sebaceous cysts in the ear canal of a gray Persian cat. The cysts appear on both the concave pinna and the ear canal. Top left and right pinnae; bottom, left and right ear canals.

Apocrine tubular glands are the major secretory glands in otitis externa. These glands increase substantially in size in response to the severity of otitis (Fig. 3–16). The sebaceous glands apparently do not proliferate in otitis externa and do not increase in size. In fact, in chronic otitis, the sebaceous glands are less active and are displaced by distended apocrine tubular glands. The apocrine tubular glands secrete their lipids and often dilute, but the total amount of cerumen produced may not increase because of the reduction in sebaceous secretions.

The secretion of the apocrine tubular glands may provide a nutrient-rich medium for microorganisms. It has been speculated that the presence of excessive apocrine tubular gland secretion coupled with the decreased sebaceous secretion in predisposed breeds facilitates growth of microorganisms. Many endocrinologic skin conditions affecting the ear stimulate the secretion of the apocrine tubular glands. Many of these same diseases are also immunosuppressive and may encourage the growth of microorganisms.

Because cerumen is a hydrophobic lipid material, excessive cerumen production associated with otitis externa provides an occlusive coating of the infected epithelial tissues. Bacteria, yeasts, proteolytic enzymes, and other vasoactive substances in exudates remain sealed under the thick

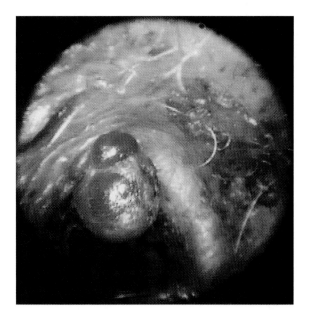

Figure 3–16

Apocrine cyst located in the vertical canal just proximal to the bend in the ear canal. This is a cystic cerumen (apocrine) gland.

lipid coating. Treatment of bacterial or yeast otitis externa must include the use of ceruminolytic flushes to remove this lipid covering, to allow the topical antimicrobial agent to contact the organisms inhabiting the infected epithelium. Ear flushes also serve to remove (1) the pro-inflammatory fatty acids produced as a result of bacterial degradation of ceruminous lipids and (2) the proteolytic enzymes released by inflammatory cells.

Once the ceruminous glands enlarge, they rarely return to pre-otitis size, and the ears produce excessive cerumen. Routine ear care must include frequent home ear flushes. Flushing the ears of affected patients to remove excessive cerumen becomes a preventive treatment. If the excessive cerumen is not removed, ceruminous otitis will result. This condition is characterized by excessive buildup of ear wax, with bacterial degradation of the lipids. The resultant free fatty acids become triggers for inflammation, leading to erythema and pruritus.

Trauma

Trauma from any external cause can affect the ears. Whether due to fight wounds, trauma to the pinna from being hit by a car, or surgical trauma, a tissue reaction triggered by a traumatic injury may lead to problems in the ear canals.

Wounds

Underlying the ear canal epithelium is a subcutaneous layer of dermis and a cylindrical to conical layer of elastic cartilage surrounded by muscles, blood vessels, and nerves. Trauma to any one of these tissues causes intense inflammation and bleeding, and may lead to acute stenosis of the ear canal from the edema that follows inflammation. In most cases, the stenosis resolves when the tissue in the damaged portion of the ear canal heals. In other cases, especially in traumatic injury to the cartilage, the healing may be very slow, and return of normal anatomical architecture incomplete. The stenotic canal that remains is the result of contracture of fibrous connective tissue or deformation of cartilage during healing. An example of the deformity of cartilage can be seen in an untreated aural hematoma in which the shape of the pinnal cartilage has been permanently changed. When the cartilaginous cylindrical shape has been compromised, the lumen of the ear canal may be obliterated. Fistulous tracts may appear around the site of facial trauma that may communicate with the ear canal (Figs. 3–17 and 3–18).

Surgical trauma from ear canal surgery can also lead to postoperative complications. Procedures such as total ear canal ablation often result in

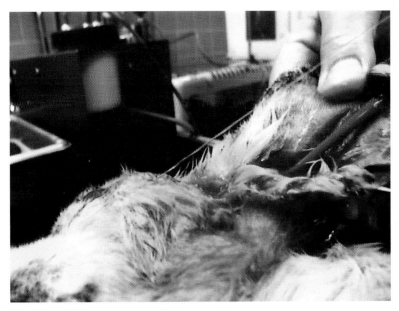

Figure 3–17

Traumatic face wound of a beagle resulted in a communication from the facial wound to the ear canal. A red rubber catheter has been placed in the ear canal, and dilute povidone-iodine is being flushed into the ear canal. As the ear canal is being flushed, the flush solution exits from the facial wound in a forceful stream parallel to the red rubber catheter.

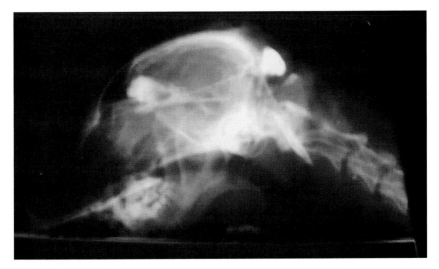

Figure 3–18

Radiograph showing infusion of iodinated contrast medium into the facial wound shown in Figure 3–17. Contrast medium can be seen filling the facial wound site, the ear canal and tympanic bulla, and the subcutaneous region in the occipital area.

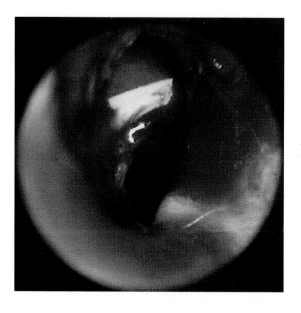

Figure 3–19

The patient, a mixed terrier, was hit by a car and had blood coming out of the ear. Examination showed that the eardrum had ruptured. The manubrium of the malleus is prominently displayed.

fistulous tracts emanating from the incompletely removed lining of the middle ear with unresolved infection. Vertical ear canal ablation or the Zepp lateral ear resection surgery requires cutting through cartilage. Suturing through cartilage incites an inflammatory reaction. Hyaluronic acid, which is released into the surrounding tissue from the cut cartilaginous matrix, stimulates intense inflammation and swelling; therefore, suturing skin to skin over the cartilage is advised.

Trauma induced by blunt force injury to the head and neck can result in a ruptured eardrum (Fig. 3–19). Fresh bleeding from the ear may be seen on examination. The ear canals in such cases must be examined for the presence of an eardrum and accumulation of blood behind the eardrum.

Trauma from Cotton-Tipped Applicators

Cotton-tipped applicators (Q-tips) are often used for removal of ear wax in humans. The dog's ear canal is long, bent, and tapered, so that the tip of an ear swab inserted into the vertical canal quickly approaches the diameter of the ear canal as it is advanced.

Trauma from the cotton-tipped applicator occurs as the ear canal is plugged by the cotton tip. The ear canal is "scraped" by the abrasive cel-

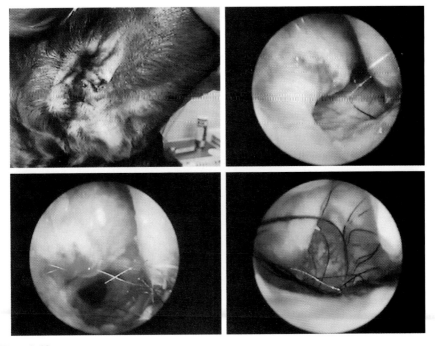

Figure 3–20

During cleaning, this ear canal became ulcerated because trauma from a cotton-tipped applicator excoriated the epithelium in the ear canal. The affected dog had *Malassezia* otitis
externa with a friable epithelial surface.

lulose or synthetic fiber. In an infected ear, the epithelium is edematous
and very often friable, so that only mild pressure from a cotton-tipped
applicator can result in ulceration (Fig. 3–20). When the ear canal
becomes ulcerated, microorganisms can flourish as growth-enhancing nu-
trients, such as blood components and serum proteins, are released into
the ear canal.

Cotton-tipped applicators also tend to push any material that may be
ahead of the cotton tip farther down the ear canal, packing cerumen into
the horizontal canal. If enough pressure is applied, this material may be
pushed right through the eardrum. Cotton-tipped applicators themselves
may perforate the eardrum if they are pushed too quickly into an ear, creating a traumatic myringotomy (Fig. 3–21).

Cotton-tipped applicators are available in a variety of tip sizes. Veterinarians should use only the small applicators in the ears of small
animals. Obtaining roll-smear cytological samples (see Chapter 2) for determining the organisms present in otic exudates can be accomplished by

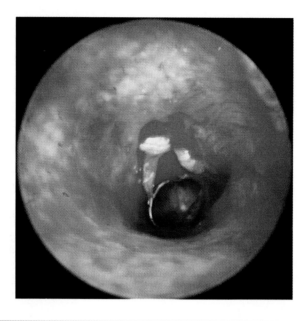

Figure 3–21

This feline ear was full of wax and debris from ear mites. Too-aggressive cleaning with a cotton-tipped applicator had ulcerated the ear canal and actually caused a perforated eardrum.

inserting the small cotton-tipped applicator into the horizontal ear canal through an otoscope cone and pulling the swab slowly along the ear canal toward the pinna.

Use of cotton-tipped applicators should be restricted to removal of liquids. The absorptive capacity of the cotton tip allows liquid to be absorbed. Simply inserting the tip very carefully into an ear filled with liquid (e.g., flush solutions, pus, mucus) while restricting movement of the applicator enables liquids to be absorbed into the tip. Repeated insertions of applicators are required until a tip is dry when removed.

Trauma from Instrumentation

Many instruments are used in the ear canal by veterinarians, groomers, and pet owners. Curettes are used to remove wax and tenacious material from the epidermal layer. Various rigid catheters are put into the ear canals for flushing and suctioning debris; sharp edges on cut urethral or feeding tubes will cut the epithelium of the ear canal. Curved hemostats are used for pulling hair from the ear canals; hemostats tend to crush tissue and, when improperly used, may cause damage to the ear canal. Water pumps, such as the Water Pik, provide a forceful stream of ear-

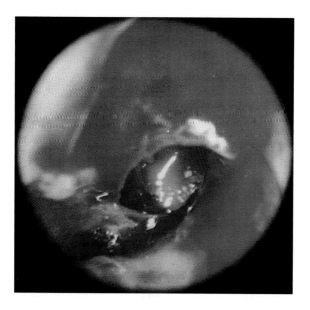

Figure 3–22

Iatrogenic traumatic myringotomy in a poodle that was put under anesthesia for ear cleaning. This large hole in the eardrum may not heal for months.

cleaning solution; increased water pressure in the ear canal can rupture an already macerated, friable eardrum.

Because most procedures done in the ear canal are performed without good visibility, trauma invariably occurs. Instruments and catheters are fairly small, and some bleeding and discomfort may be evident after the procedure. Various medications and ear cleaners may burn the ear tissue when applied. Most traumatic injuries from instruments heal rapidly. The exception is perforation of the eardrum (Fig. 3–22).

When traumatic perforation of the eardrum occurs, it is intensely painful. The patient exhibits clinical signs and pain that were not previously present. The amount of exudate in the ear canal may rapidly increase, and the otitis externa being treated appears worse. Traumatic myringotomy heals in approximately 2 to 3 weeks if iatrogenic otitis media has not been created. In the presence of an otitis externa, however, pushing exudates into the middle ear predisposes to otitis media.

Neoplasia of the Ear Canals

When a dog or cat with chronic otitis externa that does not respond to routine therapy is presented to the veterinarian, the clinician should be alerted to the possibility of a tumor or growth in the ear canal. Medical treatment for otitis externa may offer palliative relief, but the chronic recurrent nature of the disease is indicative of an underlying condition.

When cytological examination of otic exudates reveals large sheets of epithelial cells, neoplasia must be considered as a diagnosis. Chronic purulent otitis complicated by bacterial or yeast infection may also be obvious. Tumors occlude the ear canal and prevent drainage of exudate and therefore are often complicated by infection.

Symptomatology

Tumors arising in the external ear are often diagnosed only when they become large enough to be obvious. A tumor in the more distal portions of the ear canal may be obscured by wax (Fig. 3–23), or the examiner may not look past the bend in the ear canal to see a tumor in the horizontal canal. Many tumors are extremely small, and in an ear canal with a very small diameter, they predispose to infection. The tumors often have an ulcerated tip (Fig. 3–24). Occlusion of the ear canal by a tumor can cause pain and discomfort. If the patient shakes the head excessively, aural hematoma may result. It is difficult to examine the horizontal canal for tumors without an instrument such as a video otoscope (Video Vetscope, (MedRx, Inc., Seminole, FL), but if a tumor is found in the horizontal canal, it may explain the extreme discomfort the patient evidently experiences (Fig. 3–25).

Tumor of the middle ear may present as vestibular disease with head tilt or nystagmus. If visualization is possible as with a video otoscope, the tumor mass can be seen and samples taken for further diagnostic testing. Open-mouth rostro-occipital radiographs or lateral views of the tympanic bullae (Fig. 3–26) showing opacity of the osseous tympanic bulla may indicate a tumor or polyp of the middle ear. Osteolysis or fluid densities may also be seen. Computed tomography scans are also used to identify lesions within the middle ear.

Routine cleaning of the ear canal and careful examination of the skin surface of the ear canal may reveal small tumors. Good visualization and magnification are mandatory in identifying these very tiny early growths. Larger tumors may be confused with stenosis, because they are large and occlude the lumen of the ear canal. Flat tumors may look like edematous ear canals, and sessile tumors have a cobblestoned appearance (Figs. 3–27 and 3–28). Some tumors are seen only when the otoscope is placed beyond a stenotic portion of the vertical ear canal.

Secondary infection is common in ears that harbor tumor. An obstructive tumor mass allows accumulation of cerumen and debris beyond it. Because the smooth, uniform epithelial surface has been permanently changed, accumulations of wax and serum are found in the deep recesses created by the uneven surface. These crevices promote bacteria and yeast

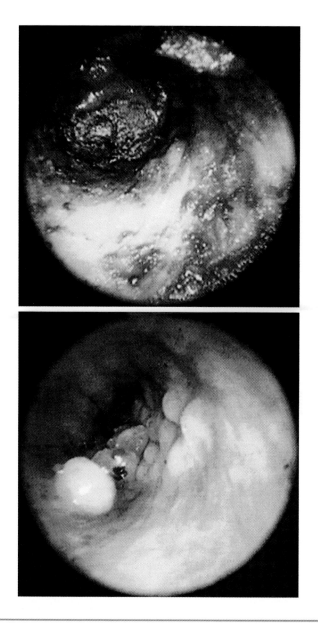

Figure 3–23

Wax accumulation in the ear canal of a schnauzer *(top)*. When the ear canal was flushed and dried, numerous cerumen gland adenomas were found *(bottom)*. Cerumen gland adenomas often are obscured by wax and may not be adequately visualized until the ear canal is cleaned.

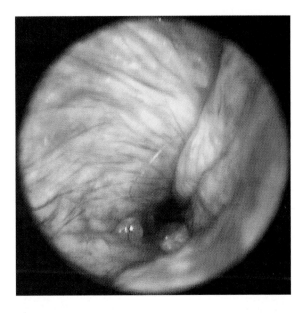

Figure 3-24

Ulcerated cerumen gland adenomas. This golden retriever had recurrent aural hematomas. The dog had been operated on three times previously for aural hematoma. When this dog was presented to the author for the fourth aural hematoma, a careful examination of the otherwise normal ear canal revealed these small ulcerated tumors. Their removal in addition to the surgery for aural hematoma cured this dog of its head shaking.

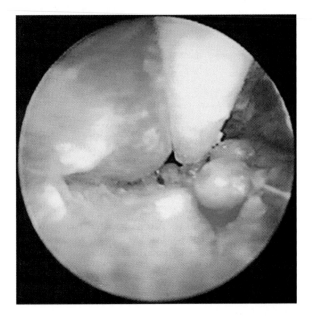

Figure 3-25

A Cocker spaniel had chronic bacterial otitis externa that would resolve with topical antibiotic/steroid drops but would recur only a few weeks after medication was stopped. A small tumor (its size can be estimated by comparing the tumor with the diameter of a tomcat catheter) with a narrow base was found. The tumor bled when manipulated and predisposed the dog to bacterial otitis and pain.

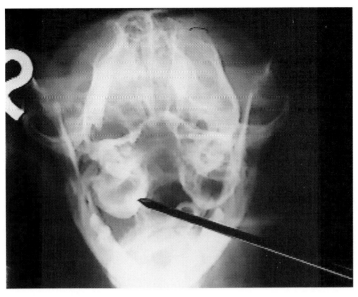

Figure 3–26

Open-mouth rostro-occipital radiograph of a cat with a unilateral nasopharyngeal polyp and otitis media. Notice the thickened tympanic bulla and the opacification of the lumen. (Courtesy of Dr. Gary Lantz, Purdue University.)

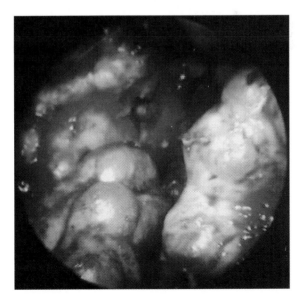

Figure 3–27

Cerumen gland adenocarcinoma has a cobblestone appearance. This tumor mass from a cat was excised by total ear canal ablation.

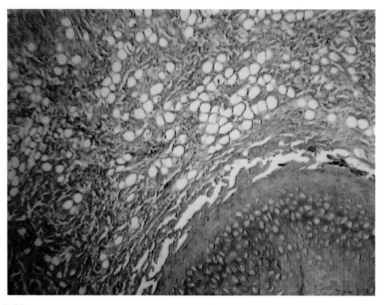

Figure 3–28

The histopathological examination of the cerumen gland adenocarcinoma in Figure 3–27 revealed numerous dilated apocrine glands extending toward the lumen from the cartilaginous base. Organic solvents used in histopathological slide preparation dissolved out the lipid material filling the ceruminous glands, leaving the tubules empty.

growth. Continued antibiotic or anti-yeast treatment is warranted in the presence of tumors because of the secondary infections and inflammation commonly associated with aural neoplasms. If the eardrum is intact, flushing the ear canal with detergent ear cleaners is beneficial to remove the cerumen and debris. If the eardrum cannot be visualized, however, caution in selecting a non-ototoxic ear cleaner is warranted.

Gross Examination

On gross examination, tumors of the ear canal can have a variety of topographical features. They may be raised (Fig. 3–29), pedunculated, broad-based, lobulated, irregular (Fig. 3–30), or ulcerated or may have a combination of these features.

For small tumors, tissue for histopathological evaluation may be obtained by curetting the tumor with a sharp-edged curette (Fig. 3–31). An endoscopic biopsy tool may be used to grasp and remove a section of tumor (Fig. 3–32). In the case of a large solitary tumor or a diffuse spreading tumor mass, a portion of the ear canal is removed surgically, and the

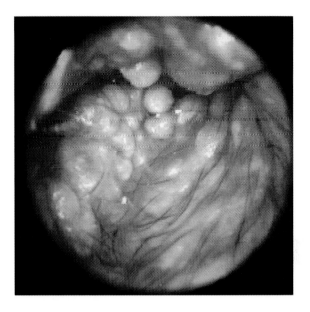

Figure 3–29

Cerumen gland adenomas in a mixed-breed dog. These raised, circular, broad-based tumors are multiple and show a variety of shapes from flat to spherical.

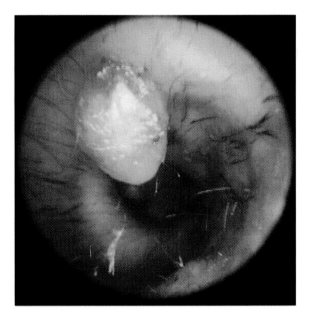

Figure 3–30

Solitary cerumen gland adenoma in the vertical ear canal of a Cocker spaniel.

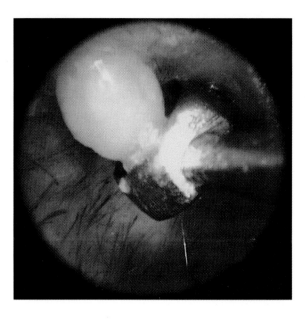

Figure 3–31

Removal of the tumor shown in Figure 3–30. A large-diameter curette with a sharp edge is placed over the tumor. The curette is then angled slightly and scraped over the base of the tumor to remove the tissue.

entire section of ear canal is submitted to the pathologist. Tissue architecture is preserved in this manner, and the pathologist can better characterize the lesion as benign or malignant. Fortunately, the circumferential cartilage of the external ear canal provides a limiting barrier to the spread of most malignant tumors. If the ear tumor and the cartilage can be submitted to the pathologist, the invasiveness of the tumor can also be determined.

Exfoliative cytological evaluation is often adequate for differentiating inflammatory from hyperplastic and neoplastic lesions. A curette is used to obtain scrapings from a suspected tumor. If the cells indicate an inflammatory lesion (neutrophils, macrophages, lymphocytes, plasma cells, and eosinophils), appropriate anti-inflammatory treatment may be instituted. If, however, clumps and clusters of large round cells are found, an epithelial neoplasm is a diagnostic possibility and the slide should be submitted to the pathologist for evaluation. Single spindle-shaped cells may indicate fibrosis or a nonepithelial type of neoplasm.

It has been theorized that chronic inflammation, more common in the dog than in the cat, may initiate progression of otic lesions from hyperplasia to dysplasia to neoplasia. It has also been speculated that bacterial degradation of the apocrine secretion from the cerumen glands that becomes inspissated in the ear canal during episodes of otitis externa may result in increased carcinogenesis. Whether the presence of a tumor leads to the chronic inflammation or chronic inflammation leads to dysplastic changes and eventually to neoplastic changes is not known.

Ear canal tumors can develop in any of the skin structures lining the ear canal, including the squamous epithelium, ceruminous or sebaceous glands, and the mesenchymal structures. Tumors arising from the external ear canal and pinna are much more common than tumors arising from the middle or inner ear.

Much controversy exists concerning the incidence of the various tumors reported in dogs and cats. Because of the difficulty in obtaining samples from the ear canal, most samples submitted to diagnostic laboratories are submitted from university or referral surgeons and not from practitioners. The number of tumors of the ear submitted for evaluation is therefore low.

Tumors of the ear canal are relatively uncommon in dogs and cats. In one report, of all tumors found in cats, only 1% to 2% were derived from aural tissue. In a second report, of all the canine aural tissue sent to different laboratories for histopathological evaluation, 2% to 6% contained tumor. Generally, tumors of the ear canal in dogs tend to be benign, and tumors of the ear canal in the cat tend to be more malignant. Fortunately, malignant neoplasms of the ear canal rarely metastasize. Failure to remove a wide en bloc section of the ear canal, however, often results in local recurrence of tumor. Total ear canal ablation may be the best surgical solution to ear neoplasia.

Most reports indicate that the benign cerumen gland adenoma is the most common tumor of the dog's ear and the malignant ceruminous gland adenocarcinoma is the most common neoplasm of the cat's ear. However, histopathological differentiation of the two types of ceruminous neoplasms is not always clear. Other benign tumors found in the ear canal of dogs are polyps, papilloma, sebaceous gland adenoma, histiocytoma, plasmacytoma, benign melanoma, and fibroma. Malignant canine neoplasms of the ear that have been reported are ceruminous gland adenocarcinomas, carcinoma of undetermined origin, squamous cell carcinoma, round cell tumor, sarcoma, malignant melanoma, and hemangiosarcoma.

Benign tumors of the cat's ear include polyp, cerumen gland adenoma, and papilloma. Malignant tumors of the cat's ear are ceruminous gland adenocarcinoma, squamous cell carcinoma, carcinoma of undetermined origin, and sebaceous gland adenocarcinoma.

Tumors found in the middle ear are rare and include fibrosarcoma (Fig. 3–33) and lymphoma.

Treatment of neoplasia found in the ear canals of dogs and cats requires surgical intervention so that the tumor mass can be completely

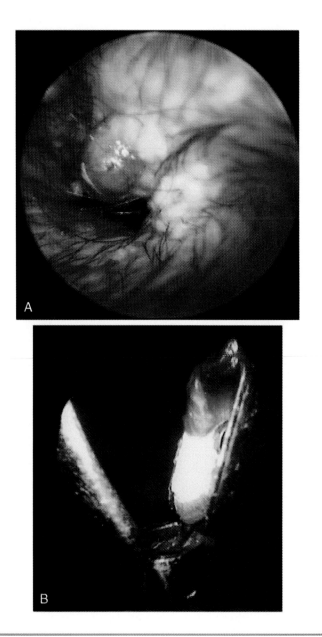

Figure 3–32

A, Large, broad-based cerumen gland tumor in the ear canal of a golden retriever. The dog had chronic *Malassezia* otitis externa. The ear canal was normal in appearance except for the tumor mass. *B,* An endoscopic biopsy tool was used through a video otoscope to take a "bite" of the tumor for histopathological evaluation.

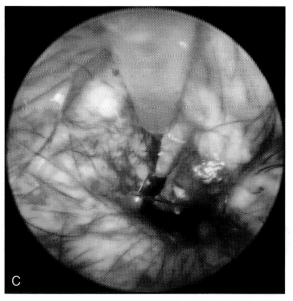

Figure 3–32 *Continued*

C, The appearance of the biopsy site after the histopathological sample was removed.

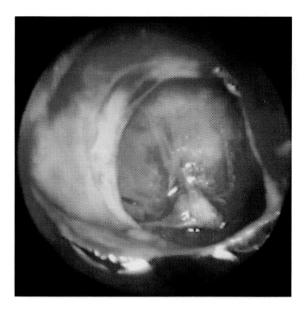

Figure 3–33

Middle ear tumor (fibrosarcoma) in a Labrador retriever mix was presented with apparent hearing loss. The eardrum of the dog was intact, but a fleshy mass was seen behind it. The other ear was considered normal. At myringotomy, the diffuse fibrosarcoma could be seen filling the tympanic bulla.

excised. Newer modalities such as electrosurgery and laser surgery through a video otoscope (Video Vetscope, MedRx, Inc., Seminole, FL) may make removal of ear canal tumors easier.

Histopathological evaluation of removed tissues helps in providing a prognosis of the disease. For malignancies, follow-up radiation therapy has been shown to be effective in preventing recurrence of many ear canal tumors.

Suggested Readings

Gotthelf LN: Secondary otitis media: An often overlooked condition. Canine Pract 20:14–20, 1995.

Logas D, Rosychuck RAW, Merchant SR: Diseases of the ear canal. Vol 24, No. 5, Vet Clin North Am Small Anim Pract. 24:905–980, 1994.

London CA, Dubilzeig RR, Vail DM, et al: Evaluation of dogs and cats with tumors of the ear canal: 145 cases (1978–1992). J Am Vet Med Assoc 208:1413–1418, 1996.

Moisan PG, Watson GL: Ceruminous gland tumors in dogs and cats: A review of 124 cases. J Am Anim Hosp Assoc 32:449–453, 1996.

Rogers KS: Tumors of the ear canal. Vet Clin North Am Small Anim Prac 18:859–868, 1988.

Theon AP, Barthez PY, Madewell BR, Griffey SM: Radiation therapy of ceruminous gland carcinomas in dogs and cats. J Am Vet Med Assoc 205:566–569, 1994.

van der Gaag I: The pathology of the external ear canal in dogs and cats. Vet Q 8:307–317, 1986.

4

Inflammatory Polyps

Louis N. Gotthelf, DVM

The inflammatory polyp may be the most common non-neoplastic growth found in the ears of cats. There appears to be no breed, gender, or age predilection for polyps in cats. Inflammatory polyps are most often found in the young mature cat, suggesting a congenital origin. Some cats are presented to the veterinarian with waxy accumulations deep in the ear canal at the level of the eardrum (Fig. 4–1). Other cats are presented with a severe mucopurulent exudate in the ear canal resulting from otitis media.

Otoscopic examination reveals a pink to red, fleshy mass deep in the ear canal. When the mass can be seen in the external ear canal, it has already protruded through the eardrum, having ruptured it as the polyp grew. Otitis media is usually found concurrently in the cat with an inflammatory polyp that has grown from the middle ear into the external ear canal.

The inflammatory polyp is also called a nasopharyngeal polyp. Polyps originate in either the eustachian tube or the tympanic bulla; however, most polyps in cats seem to originate from the middle ear mucosa. Polyps originating in the eustachian tube may not be present in the middle ear or ear canal at all but can be found protruding from the external opening of the eustachian tube on the lateral wall of the nasopharynx. The location of the polyp in the nasopharynx may be found by retracting the soft

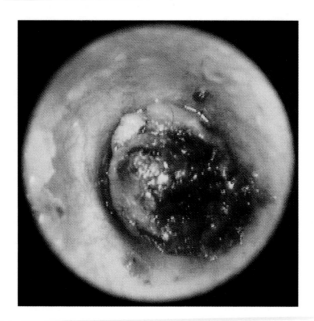

Figure 4–1

Waxy accumulation in the ear canal of a cat. This mass was located deep in the horizontal portion of the ear canal. The cat was presented for head tilt and ataxia.

palate rostrally. The cat with an oropharyngeal polyp shows respiratory symptoms, such as stertorous respiration, voice changes, wheezing, dyspnea, and dysphagia.

Otitis media in cats may result from ascending infection from the nasopharynx through the auditory tube. Otitis media in most cats and dogs, however, results from extension of external ear canal disease through a ruptured eardrum.

Inflammatory polyps predispose the ear to otitis externa and otitis media. The polyp mass enlarges to fill the bony cavity of the tympanic bulla and then grows through the eardrum and ruptures it. As a result, bacteria, yeasts, and ear mites residing in the external ear canal are allowed access to the respiratory epithelium of the tympanic bulla of the middle ear, leading to otitis media. As the polyp enlarges, it rapidly approaches the diameter of the ear canal. The polyp acts to seal the ear canal, so that exudates from otitis media are trapped behind the polyp in the middle ear.

Clinical Presentation

The predominant clinical signs in the cat with an inflammatory polyp of the ear canal are discharge from the ear canal and head shaking or head tilt. Nystagmus and vestibular disease may be present in more severe cases. Careful flushing of the ear canal and removal of exudates promote good visualization with a video otoscope (Video Vetscope, MedRx, Seminole, FL). Examination reveals a fleshy mass occluding the ear canal and tympanic bulla (Fig. 4–2). If the mass can be moved while grasped with an endoscopic forceps, it is not attached to the ear canal epithelium. In most cases, as the polyp is moved, the mass that was obstructing the middle ear allows exudates trapped in the middle ear to escape, filling the external ear canal.

Pathogenesis

Just why polyps develop remains a mystery. Viruses and bacteria have been implicated. Whether otitis media is primary or secondary in the pathogenesis of polyps is also unknown. Experimentally, polyps have been induced in rats by placing type 3 pneumococci into the middle ear cavity. In only 44% of the rats in this study did a polyp develop in the infected ear. None of the rats had a polyp in the untreated ear.

Polyps are inflammatory lesions that arise in response to chronic irritation of the mucosa. It is theorized that the events leading to polyp formation are (1) localized rupture of the respiratory epithelium lining the

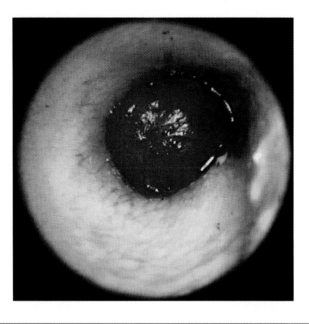

Figure 4–2

Nasopharyngeal polyp occluding the ear canal of a cat. The waxy accumulation shown in Figure 4–1 was removed to reveal this red, fleshy mass in the cat's ear canal.

tympanic bulla or eustachian tube followed by (2) luminal protrusion of the lamina propria through the epithelial defect and re-epithelialization of the protruded tissue. As the epithelium covering the polyp becomes damaged by infection or by physical trauma from its own movement against surrounding tissue, this process repeats a number of times, resulting in significant production of fibrous stroma and enlargement of the mass.

Histologic Features

Histologically, polyps are hyperplastic inflammatory proliferations of middle ear mucosa. They are composed of a well-vascularized fibrous tissue stroma covered with respiratory epithelium. The stroma is edematous, and the submucosa contains a mixed population of acute and chronic inflammatory cells, including neutrophils, macrophages, and plasma cells. Variable amounts of lymphocytes may also be present. It is difficult to determine the exact point of origin of a polyp histologically because the respiratory epithelium of the mucous membrane in the tympanic cavity, auditory tube, and nasopharynx is continuous.

Removal and Follow-up Therapy

Polyps are generally pedunculated—that is, attached to the mucosa by a thin stalk (Fig. 4–3). Removal of the stalk is essential to prevent recurrence of the lesion. If there is radiographic evidence of involvement of the tympanic bulla, a lateral (Fig 4 4) or ventral bulla osteotomy with careful curettage of the mucosal origin of the polyp is performed.

A common method for removal of a polyp is to grasp the polyp with an alligator forceps and apply gentle traction. The polyp may be rotated 90 degrees, and the surgeon should have a good grasp of the mass. A quick tug on the forceps then causes the thin vascular peduncle or stalk to break, enabling the mass to be removed intact (Fig. 4–5). Traction is preferred to excision because it is more likely to remove the peduncle. When the stalk of the polyp is excised, the blood supply from the submucosa remains intact (Fig. 4–6). When the stalk is stretched by gentle traction, the vascular supply to the polyp is destroyed, and regrowth is unlikely.

The author has removed many intact polyps from dogs and cats in this manner. The use of a video otoscope allows excellent visualization of the polyp. It is simple to use the endoscopic grasping forceps to obtain a good grasp of the mass while watching the magnified image on the video

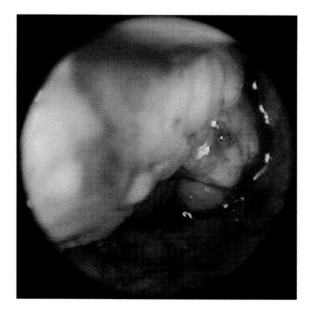

Figure 4–3

Nasopharyngeal polyp in a dog. The long stalk or peduncle in this polyp extended from the middle ear mucosa through the ear canal. The actual polyp mass was located at the pinnal opening of the ear canal (see Figure 4–7).

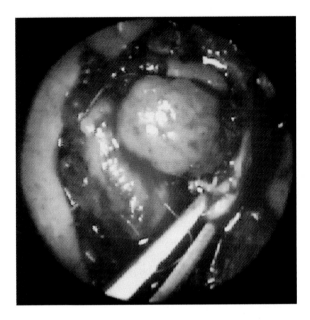

Figure 4–4

Lateral bulla osteotomy. When the polyp is inaccessible from the ear canal, an open procedure is required to excise the mass. In this cat, the polyp was not visible through the otoscope owing to a stenotic condition in the vertical ear canal (a tumor) but was found during a total ear canal ablation.

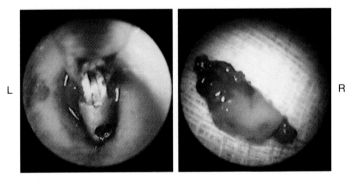

L   R

Figure 4–5

Removal of a polyp using a video otoscope. *Left,* Under direct video visualization, the polyp mass is grabbed with an endoscopic grasping forceps and rotated. *Right,* Then a quick jerk on the forceps breaks the peduncle, and the polyp is removed intact.

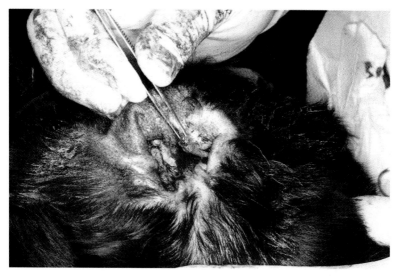

Figure 4–6

When the polyp is removed by excision, the peduncle remains (grasped in thumb forceps). Unless this vascular supply is removed at the time of surgery, the polyp will probably grow back.

monitor. Without adequate visualization, only a portion of the polyp may be removed; in this case, regrowth may be rapid and clinical signs associated with polyp will return.

Polyps occur in dogs much less often than in cats, but the polyps found in dogs tend to grow much larger, often extending from the middle ear into the vertical ear canal and pinna (Fig. 4–7). In one report, a canine nasopharyngeal polyp localized in the nasopharynx was so large that an incision in the soft palate was required to access it at the external opening of the auditory tube in order to grasp and remove it.

After removal of the mass, topical corticosteroid solution is infused directly onto the tympanic bulla mucosal surface. This is accomplished by placing a tomcat catheter into the bulla through the 2-mm channel of the video otoscope and infusing the corticosteroid solution onto the mucous membrane lining from a syringe attached to the catheter. Treatment for specific factors perpetuating concurrent otitis externa or otitis media, such as ear mite infestation and bacterial or yeast infections, must also continue.

It has been reported that one third of all polyps recur after partial removal, so it is important to remove the mass by the stalk. Clients should understand that there is a possibility of regrowth so that recheck visits to look for new polyp growth are needed.

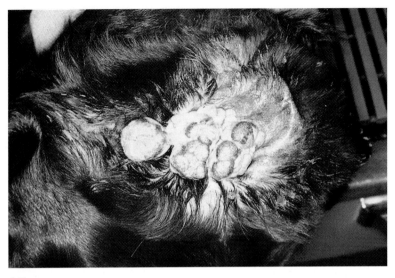

Figure 4–7

Canine inflammatory polyp. The patient, a Labrador retriever, was presented with both pinnae extending laterally from the head. Inflammatory polyps were present in both ears. The white polyp mass visible in this photograph filled the external opening to the ear canal. As it grew, the polyp had molded to the epithelial folds of the tragus of the pinna but was easily separated from the pinna. Each had a thick vascular stalk that extended through the entire ear canal to the middle ear (see Figure 4–3). The polyps were easily removed by excision, and the stalks were removed with traction.

Suggested Readings

Boothe HW: Surgery of the tympanic bulla (otitis media and nasopharyngeal polyps). Probl Vet Med 3:254–269, 1991.

Fingland RB, Gratzek A, Vorhies MW, Kirpensteijn J: Nasopharyngeal polyp in a dog. J Am Anim Hosp Assoc 29:311–314, 1993.

5

Primary Causes
of Ear Disease

Louis N. Gotthelf, DVM

Primary causes of ear disease are:

- Hypersensitivity diseases (see Chapter 6)
- Parasites found in the ear canal
- Keratinization and glandular disorders
- Foreign bodies that gain access to the ear canal, including sand, dirt, and dried medications placed in the ear canal

Parasites

Ear Mites

Ear mites are the most common parasites found in the ear canal of dogs and cats. *Otodectes cyanotis,* the ear mite, has been identified in a number of animal species, both domestic and wild. A nonburrowing psoroptid mite, the ear mite feeds on epithelial cells, lymph, and blood. In dogs and cats, ear mites can cause a severely pruritic parasitic otitis that is commonly complicated by secondary bacterial infection, otitis media, and, in cats, a systemic hypersensitivity reaction.

A patient affected with ear mites shakes the head violently and scratches at the ears. Facial abrasions and hair loss may be evident in the area between the lateral canthus of the eyelid and the ear. When examined, the ear canals display the reddish brown to black, dried crusty exudate typically found in ear mite infections. The brown color is presumed to be from blood. On otoscopic examination, the mites can be seen as white insects crawling on the surface of the exudate (Fig. 5–1).

If the otoscope cone is held very steady, the mite activity increases, because the light arouses the mites and makes them more active. When viewed with a video otoscope (Video Vetscope, MedRx, Inc., Seminole, FL), which has high magnification and a bright light source, the mites can often be seen in colonies, with thousands of scurrying mites in each otoscopic field.

In some cases, especially in dogs, only a few mites may be inhabiting the ear canal (Fig. 5–2). They often elude otoscopic or microscopic detection. It has been theorized that either severe inflammation in the ear drives out the mites or the exudates destroy them. The severity of the symptoms associated with *Otodectes* may be due to the Arthus-like hypersensitivity reaction provoked by the presence of a very few mites.

One useful technique for diagnosing ear mite infection in patients in which *Otodectes* is suspected but mites are not seen otoscopically is a roll smear. A small cotton-tipped applicator is saturated with mineral oil and used to swab the ear canal. The cotton tip of the applicator is placed in a drop of mineral oil on a microscope slide, and the tip is rolled back and

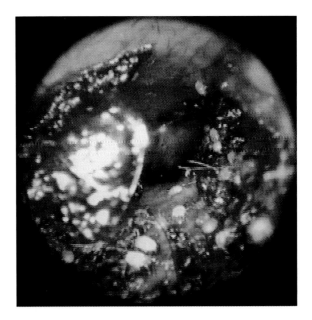

Figure 5–1

Ear mites in a cat. The ear mites *(Otodectes cyanotis)* can be seen as small white insects crawling on the surface of the typical dry, flaky dark crusts commonly found in ear mite–infested ears.

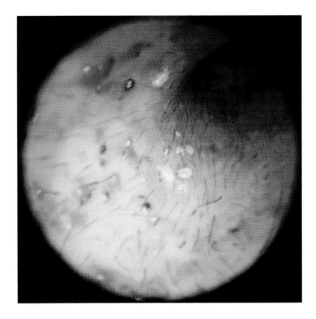

Figure 5–2

Ear mites in an 8-week-old puppy. Only a few mites are present, but they caused a severe pruritus. The puppy was scratching its ears and shaking its head.

forth to move most of the harvested material from the cotton tip to the slide. The slide is then cover-slipped and examined under low-power (40×) magnification. Adult mites, often duos representing breeding pairs, can usually be seen crawling through the field. Alternatively, the typical long, oval eggs of *Otodectes* may instead be the only evidence of infection (see Fig. 2–22).

The ear mite lives primarily in the ear, where it feeds on epithelial tissue and blood. Female *Otodectes* mites lay solitary eggs in the ear canal, and within 2 to 3 weeks of maturation, adult mites begin feeding. Ear mites are prolific; in a short time, mite infestation may be severe.

Although ear mites can live in the environment, direct transmission of *Otodectes* from animal to animal is accepted as the usual mode of transmission. Mites may jump onto any part of the animal's body and migrate into the ear canal. Many affected 6-week-old kittens have severe ear disease because they acquired *Otodectes* from their queens during the neonatal period. In situations of high animal density, such as shelters, pet shops, and breeding colonies, ear mites can affect the entire population. It is rare for a solitary indoor cat to acquire ear mites.

The aggressive epithelial feeding habits of *Otodectes* cause damage to the epithelium of the external ear canal. Secondary bacterial infection may result from the loss of the epithelial protective barrier in the ear canal; a contributing factor is the high serum protein substrates that are made available as a result. Ear mites at the eardrum can actually chew their way through the thin tympanic membrane (Fig. 5–3). The middle ear epithelium is then exposed to *Otodectes*. When the mites feed in the middle ear, punctures in the respiratory epithelium and the resultant inflammation may be a stimulus for polyp formation.

Ear Mites in Cats

A unique result of *Otodectes* infestation in the cat is a systemic hypersensitivity reaction. Mite antigens gain access to the blood as the mites feed and denude the epithelium. Experimentally infected cats showed an immediate hypersensitivity reaction to an intradermal mite extract. Cats infected for 35 days showed an Arthus (type III) reaction. Serum-precipitating antibodies were noted at 45 days after infection.

If a cat has ear mites but not pruritus, the animal is probably not allergic to the mites. However, severely pruritic cats are probably hypersensitive. Cats presented with the classic signs of miliary dermatitis (papular crusts around the neck, dorsolumbar area, and inguinal region) should be treated systemically for *Otodectes* as part of the treatment for pruritus. In these hypersensitive cases, systemic corticosteroids such as methylprednisolone acetate (Depo-Medrol, Upjohn Pharmacia) may also be needed to control the pruritus.

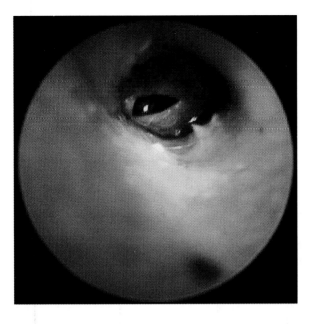

Figure 5–3

Ruptured tympanic membrane seen after instillation of an ear flush solution into a cat's ear. The cat was severely affected with ear mites and had a mucopurulent discharge when presented to the veterinarian. The eardrum is ruptured and edematous.

Treatment

Treatment of *Otodectes* has traditionally involved the use of ear drops containing a variety of ingredients. Thorough cleaning of the ear canal with the patient sedated prior to the use of any topical medication hastens the therapeutic effects of the topical medication. All ear mite medications contain insecticides, which are placed in the ear canal to kill the mites. Additional ingredients are compounded in these topicals, including (1) ceruminolytics to loosen the inspissated ceruminous material, (2) antibiotics to treat the secondary bacterial infection, and (3) mineral oil, which is used as a vehicle to float the debris to the pinnal surface so it can be removed. Mineral oil may also have the beneficial effect of blocking the breathing tubes of the mites and suffocating them. Drops for ear mite infections need to be used for at least 14 days so that the mites hatching from eggs in the canal are killed before the life cycle starts over. Retreatment at monthly intervals has been recommended for free-roaming cats with chronic mite infestations.

Because the anthelminthic ivermectin has been demonstrated to be a good acaricide as well, it has been used for treatment of ear mites in dogs and cats. Ivermectin is approved for use in dogs and cats only as a heartworm preventative. Injectible ivermectin (Ivomec 1% Injection, Merial, Ltd.) is used at a dose of 250 μg/kg or 0.1 mL/10 lb of body weight. It is injected subcutaneously every 10 days to 2 weeks for 2 or 3 injections. Because it is now well established that ear mites also live on the skin, the injections serve to treat the entire body. All contact animals in the environment should be treated concurrently. Ivermectin can be placed directly into each ear canal as a topical treatment for ear mites or placed on the skin over the dorsum of the cat, at a dose of 0.5 mg/kg every 2 weeks for 2 to 3 applications.

Some severe neurological reactions and even deaths have been reported in cats treated with injections of ivermectin. Kittens treated with doses that exceed 250 μg/kg may be more susceptible to the fatal reactions than adult cats. The reason may be linked to the age at which the blood-brain barrier develops in kittens. It is hypothesized that without an adequately mature blood-brain barrier, ivermectin may gain access to the brain in the affected kittens and interact with gamma-aminobutyric acid (GABA) receptors, causing neurological signs to develop.

Fipronil (Frontline TopSpot, Merial, Ltd.), a monthly flea control insecticide, has demonstrated miticidal activity in both dogs and cats. Because many animals in flea-infested areas are being treated with fipronil for control of fleas, *Otodectes* control is a beneficial feature of this product. Fipronil-treated pets that roam may acquire *Otodectes* mites on their skin, but the mites will be killed prior to reproducing; this may act as a preventative against ear mites.

Treatment for otitis externa secondary to *Otodectes* infection must not be overlooked. Antibiotic and antibiotic-corticosteroid ear drops are used until the epithelial surface heals. If otitis media is present, the ear canal and tympanic bulla should be flushed and suctioned carefully to remove any debris that may have gained access to the tympanic bulla.

Demodex Mites

Occasionally, *Demodex* mites may be found on a mineral oil swab from the ear of a dog with otitis (Fig. 5–4). Amitraz in mineral oil administered daily in the ear works well to decrease this mite population.

Fleas and Ticks

Fleas sometimes crawl into the external ear canal and feed (Fig. 5–5). Flea allergy dermatitis rarely has an effect on the ear, however. Fleas crawling around the ears of cats seem to cause a cutaneous sensitivity, and cats scratch at their ears. Ticks may attach to the ear canal epithelium and cartilage, resulting in a very painful ear (Fig. 5–6). Thorough

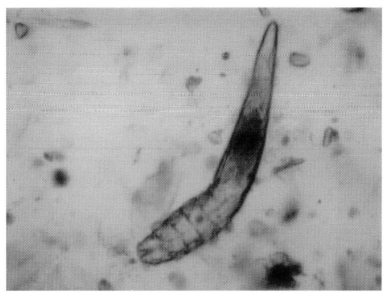

Figure 5–4

A *Demodex* mite was found on this mineral oil swab taken from the stenotic ear canal of an 8-year-old Cocker spaniel. No active areas of *Demodex* mange were found on the dog's skin.

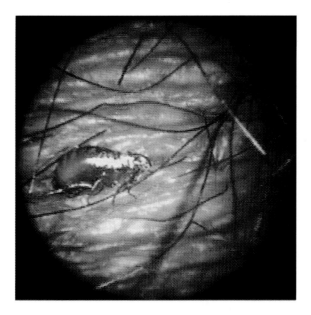

Figure 5–5

Occasionally, fleas are found in and around the ears. Fleas that crawl around the ears of a cat cause behaviors suggestive of an ear infection even though the ear is perfectly normal.

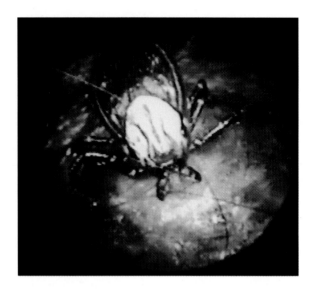

Figure 5–6

Brown dog tick *(Ripicephalus sanguineous)* on the ear of a dog. An area of inflammation surrounds the insertion of the tick's mouth parts, which can be very painful to the dog.

examination of tick-infested dogs should include a careful examination of the epithelial folds of the tragus.

Keratinization Disorders

Primary idiopathic seborrhea, hypothyroidism, and sex hormone imbalances can be inciting causes of ear disease (see Chapter 12).

Hypothyroidism is the most common hormone imbalance found in dogs. It is responsible for many changes in the skin of the ear canal that allow colonization by secondary invaders such as bacteria and yeasts. Lymphocytic thyroiditis is the most common cause of hypothyroidism in dogs. It has been postulated that this condition is a progressive disease that starts at a young age and progresses to destruction of thyroid parenchyma. When thyroid production is significantly impaired by fibrosis, the clinical signs of hypothyroidism begin to appear. As the disease process continues, destruction of the thyroid gland proceeds until the thyroid tissue is replaced with fibrosis.

Thyroglobulin assays may be useful in determining which patients may be at risk for developing hypothyroidism due to lymphocytic thyroiditis. Even before serum thyroxine levels begin to fall, and prior to the onset of clinical disease, the destruction of the thyroid follicles results in increased levels of thyroglobulin.

Discussions of thyroid hormone assays and interpretation of test results can be found in numerous internal medicine and endocrinology references. The current standard of thyroxine measurement is determination of free thyroxine (T_4) by equilibrium dialysis (fT_4) or of total T_4 (tT_4). An increased thyroid-stimulating hormone (TSH) level, coupled with a low or borderline T_4 level, is often used to separate thyroidal from nonthyroidal illness.

Clinically, hypothyroidism is often misdiagnosed because of the influence of other nonthyroidal factors on results of thyroid function tests. Many dogs with low serum thyroxine levels are not truly hypothyroid. Dogs that are being treated with corticosteroids or sulfa drugs may have a low T_4 level and yet be euthyroid, as confirmed by a normal TSH level. When a dog is truly hypothyroid, the T_4 level is low and the TSH value is elevated. Response to thyroxine supplementation is dramatic.

Certain breeds seem to be predisposed to hypothyroidism and also seem to pose the greatest challenge to the veterinarian dealing with their otitis externa. Shar Pei, poodle, Cocker spaniel, golden retriever, chow chow, and German shepherd seem to be hypothyroid-prone breeds in which otitis externa is frequently a feature of the hypothyroid condition.

In the ear, lowered thyroid hormone alters the fatty acid composition of the lipids in the cerumen. When the dog is hypothyroid, the cerumen glands may become overactivated, resulting in ceruminous otitis. On cytologic examination, few organisms are found, but the predominance of keratinocytes along with the presence of nonstaining sebaceous cellular debris is common.

Hypothyroidism results in seborrheic dermatitis. *Malassezia* colonizes the skin and ears because of the greater availability of lipid substrates utilized by *Malassezia*. Often the first sign of hypothyroidism is the intense pruritus due to *Malassezia* in a dog with ceruminous otitis externa. *Malassezia* then induces profound epidermal changes in the already altered ear canal, complicating the seborrheic condition and increasing patient discomfort.

Low circulating thyroid hormone levels also are associated with decreased activity of B and T lymphocytes in the skin, diminishing the ability of the skin to respond to cutaneous bacteria. The effect of this condition in concert with that of the altered lipid layer is that staphylococci normally held in check by these immunological mechanisms colonize the skin, resulting in pyoderma. Bacterial otitis externa, usually involving staphylococci, results.

Proper diagnosis and treatment of hypothyroidism involve removal of the primary cause of the otitis externa. Treatment for the secondary infection due to bacteria or yeasts reduces the perpetuating inflammatory reaction.

Even after hypothyroidism is controlled, the cerumen glands continue to secrete large amounts of altered lipids. Ceruminolytics and frequent ear flushing help prevent recurrence of the secondary infections caused by the pathological changes induced in the ear canal.

Foreign Bodies

Patients presented with ear disease may have acquired foreign material in their ears that contribute to otitis. A number of ear medications are composed of oils and particulate drying agents that may not be removed by the normal epithelial clearance mechanism. These hardened medications remain in contact with the ear canal epithelium (Fig. 5–7). The ear canal may be occluded by these concretions, resulting in otitis media. When they are identified, these concretions may be gently flushed out of the ear canal with warm flush solution and pressure. They may also be curetted from the canal or grasped with an alligator forceps.

Frequently, plant awns and foxtails get into the ear canal. They are conical, and their narrow base is fairly smooth and round, so entrance into the ear canal is relatively easy. However, the other end of a plant awn

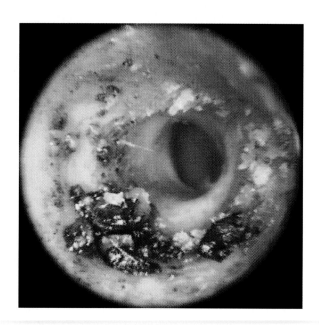

Figure 5–7

A neomycin-containing powder was used in the ear of this cat. The white powder can be seen adherent to the cerumen on the lining of the ear canal.

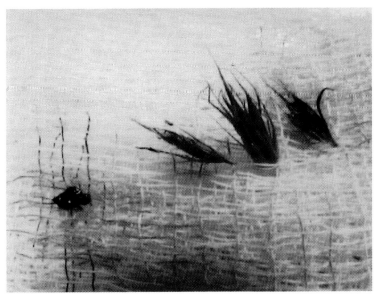

Figure 5–8

Plant awns retrieved from a Cocker spaniel with severe mucopurulent otic discharge. A large, sticky, odoriferous hair mat was found around the opening of the external ear canal. The plant awns had migrated through the eardrum, initiating an otitis media. The unkempt dog's coat was also filled with plant material.

has a sharp radiating crown of spikes (Fig. 5–8). Movement of the awn out of the ear canal is prevented because the diameter of the clump of radiating spikes tends to increase with that outward directional movement. The awns migrate one way—deep into the ear canal—and gain access to the middle ear through a ruptured eardrum. Significant otitis media results. The ear canals frequently fill with copious exudate, and the awns are difficult to visualize. Good cleaning of the ear canal aids in identifying plant material in the ear canal.

A video otoscope helps facilitate the removal of plant awns and foxtails. Such an instrument allows clear visualization and good light for identification. The grasping forceps can be inserted through the working channel of the instrument so that the awn or foxtail can be removed. Gentle traction on the plant material collapses the radial spikes and allows its easy removal from the bulla or ear canal.

6

Factors That Perpetuate Otitis Externa

Louis N. Gotthelf, DVM

O titis externa is a common malady, occurring in 15% to 20% of dogs and 4% to 7% of cats in a veterinary practice. Otitis externa is also one of the most frustrating diseases for veterinarians and owners to treat effectively. Treatment regimens vary widely, and a myriad of products containing a variety of ingredients are available for the treatment of ear disease.

Effective treatment of otitis externa often varies from one patient to another and is a challenge to the veterinarian. Treatments successful in one patient may not help in the next. Each patient and each ear must be considered individually and treatment regimens must be tailored to the specific case.

Dermatological conditions often affect the ear canal, making it susceptible to otitis externa. The ear canal is an invagination of epidermis forming a hollow skin tube inside the head that ends at the eardrum. Pathological mechanisms affecting the skin of the animal also affect the epithelial tube lining the ear canal. For example, a dog with atopy may also show inflammation of the ear canal resulting in redness, swelling, heat, and pain (Fig. 6–1). In a cylindrical tube such as the ear canal, inflammation decreases the lumen diameter, tending to reduce both the

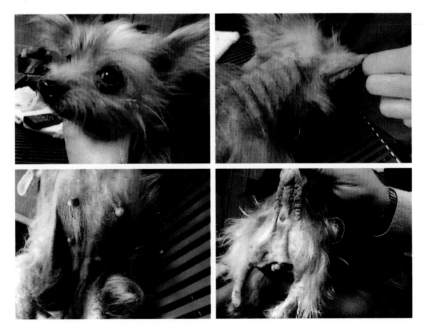

Figure 6–1

Underlying skin disease predisposes the ear to inflammation and secondary bacterial or yeast infection. The patient, a 5-year-old Yorkshire terrier with severe allergic skin disease complicated by *Malassezia* dermatitis, also had severe *Malassezia* otitis externa.

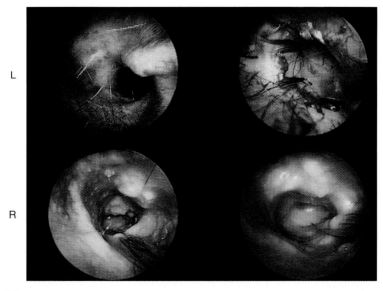

L

R

Figure 6–2

Left and right ear canals from a dog with atopy. *Top,* The left ear canal *(left)* and eardrum *(right)* are normal. *Bottom,* The right ear canal *(left)* is severely inflamed with a thick exudate that has drained into the horizontal ear canal. Cytological examination revealed *Pseudomonas,* and when the ear canal was flushed, there was no eardrum. The infection had moved into the middle ear, resulting in otitis media. Hyposensitization allowed complete resolution of the dog's otitis.

ventilation and drying of the ear canal. Without ventilation, the humidity level of the ear canal rises, a factor favorable for bacterial growth.

Papules, pustules, crusts, ulcers, and alopecia that may occur on the skin of the trunk may also occur on the skin of the ear canal. Because the ear canal is L-shaped, exudates from these lesions tend to accumulate in the horizontal portion of the ear canal (Fig. 6–2). In the treatment of skin disease, shampoo therapy utilizing a variety of compounds formulated for specific purposes acts to remove irritating substances and improve healing. In the ear canal, ear flushing solutions containing a variety of ingredients are also used for adjunctive therapy of diseases of the ear canal.

New approaches to the medical management of otitis externa in dogs and cats have now been introduced. They include (1) cytological evaluation of exudate to identify disease processes and to determine the type of disease organisms that may be present, (2) flushing products to remove exudates and to disinfect the canal epithelium, and (3) elucidations of pathophysiological mechanisms showing that otitis externa is a secondary manifestation of underlying skin disease. New combinations of topical medications have been formulated to be effective against bacteria,

fungi, and inflammation. The fluoroquinolone antibiotics, injectible ivermectin, and topical fipronil for ear mite infestations have reduced the use
of potentially ototoxic antibiotics, oils, and insecticides in the ear canal.

Cytological Evaluation

The first step in approaching ear disease is to examine a cytological
preparation of the otic exudate. Obtaining samples and preparing a slide
to examine constitute a simple procedure that should be a part of the
minimum approach to every case of otitis presented to the veterinarian. A
sample is obtained with the use of a small cotton-tipped applicator. The
swab is inserted through a disinfected otoscope cone positioned near the
horizontal canal. The swab is extended beyond the plastic cone, and pressure is applied to the ear canal epithelium as the swab is drawn back
through the cone. Every attempt is made to sample from the horizontal
canal epithelium only, because the vertical canal is often contaminated
with a number of commensal organisms unrelated to the ear disease.

The material collected on the swab is rolled onto a clean microscope
slide, with the exudate from the left ear on the left part of the slide and the
sample from the right ear on the right side. The slide is appropriately
labeled with the patient's name, the date of the collection, and which
sample is from which ear (see Fig. 2–18). It is then heat fixed and stained
with a modified Wright's blood stain. A drop of slide-mounting medium is
placed over the dried, stained material. Then a coverslip is placed on top of
the drop, and the glue is allowed to set. The use of slide-mounting medium
makes a permanent record of the cytological characteristics, which can be
stored for comparison at subsequent examinations. Alternatively, immer-
sion oil can be smeared along the stained slide and examined.

Examination of the slide under low-power magnification allows an
overall view of the cellular debris. High-power examination can help
identify and quantify organisms. Cytological evaluation is very helpful in
detecting bacteria and yeasts responsible for secondary infection. Normal
commensal bacteria may be found, but in otitis, abnormal increases in
numbers of organisms to the point of almost a pure culture, the presence
of neutrophils, or both indicate secondary bacterial infection. Often only
one ear is affected clinically, but the same organism may be found in the
unaffected ear. Sometimes each ear of the same animal has a different organism and needs a different treatment. The severity of the otitis may
also be different in the two ears.

When infectious organisms are seen under high-power (400×) magnification, cocci are usually *Staphylococcus,* and rods are usually
Pseudomonas or *Proteus* (Fig. 6–3). Budding yeasts of *Malassezia* may be
seen individually in the background on a roll smear (Fig. 6–4), but large

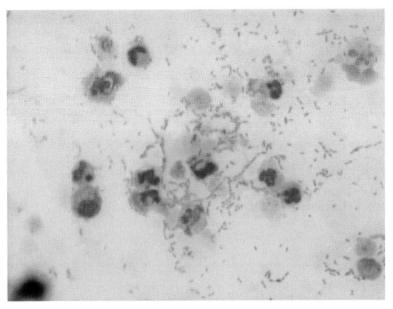

Figure 6–3

Cytological preparation from an infected ear revealed a large number of rods and neutrophils. Rods are usually *Pseudomonas* or *Proteus*. Neutrophils indicate an inflammatory process.

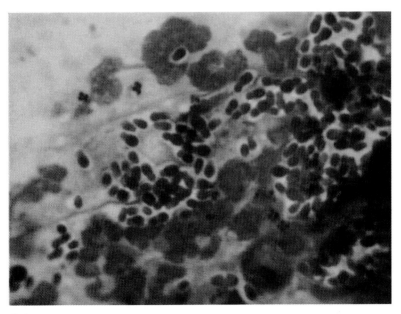

Figure 6–4

Malassezia organisms are readily identified from the large budding yeasts seen on this stained roll smear of otic exudate.

numbers of yeasts colonizing on exfoliated epithelium indicate secondary yeast infection. *Staphylococcus* and *Malassezia* are often found together in the same ear, and there is evidence to suggest that *Malassezia* growth is stimulated by *Staphylococcus.*

Bacterial culture and sensitivity testing of exudates may be useful in cases of resistant otitis externa. Many organisms have developed resistance to the routinely used antibiotics, and they should be identified. A limitation of bacterial sensitivity testing is that the organism's sensitivity or resistance is reported by the laboratory on the basis of the minimum inhibitory concentration (MIC) of the antibiotic in the blood required to kill the bacteria. Topical antibiotics can achieve significantly higher concentrations in the ear canal than systemic antibiotics can in the blood. The high topical antibiotic concentration may actually be effective at killing a bacterium that was reported as resistant. Samples for culture should be taken from the horizontal canal if possible so that contaminant bacteria are not mistaken for the offending organism. Routine culture of exudate in all cases of otitis is often unrewarding and extremely misleading because four or five bacterial isolates are often reported.

Roll smear cytological evaluation becomes useful in determining the etiology of those cases of otitis externa without secondary infection. Sheets of epithelial cells may indicate neoplasia as the cause of otitis externa, and the presence of numerous intact nonstaining epithelial cells may indicate a seborrheic condition. Parasites such as *Otodectes* and *Demodex,* which may be present in the ceruminous exudate, may be found on cytological preparations, but these parasites are better viewed on a direct mineral oil preparation; this type of preparation is made by rolling the ear swab sample in a drop of mineral oil on a slide.

Flushing of the Ear Canal

After the class of disease and the type of infection are determined, the next step is to sedate or anesthetize the animal so that a thorough flushing and suctioning of the ear canal can be done. It is imperative that exudates and dried medications that have accumulated in the ear canal be removed so that the canal epithelium itself can be evaluated. Good visualization of the ear canal after flushing helps to ensure that the vertical and horizontal canals are clean and free of debris. The efficacy of otic medications is enhanced when they are applied directly onto the cleaned epithelial surface.

Care must be taken in the selection of a flushing agent, because so many ear cleaners contain materials that are potentially ototoxic when the eardrum is not intact (see Chapter 9). Prior to using an ear cleaner, the veterinarian should read the label to see whether it can be used when the eardrum is damaged. Many manufacturers are now placing a warning about this issue on their labels.

Warmed saline or warmed, very dilute povidone-iodine solutions (*not* iodine *scrub,* which contains detergents) are safe flushing materials to use. A Water Pik can be used to loosen the exudate, but the pressure in such an instrument can be very high, necessitating extra caution to avoid rupturing the eardrum. Ear curettes, designed to remove debris firmly attached to the epithelium, are useful for scraping the ear canal to dislodge large pieces of wax and epithelial shreds. Curettes are also useful for harvesting cells for cytological evaluation when a tumor mass is suspected.

After the external ear canal is flushed, it is cleaned with a catheter attached to suction. With good visualization, small pieces of wax, epithelial flakes, and foreign material can be removed. Flushing and suctioning may need to be repeated several times to ensure that the ear canal is thoroughly cleaned.

Cotton-tipped applicators should *never* be used to clean ears! When a cotton-tipped applicator is pushed into an ear canal full of exudate, the exudate is pushed farther toward the eardrum, making cleaning more difficult and possibly rupturing a weakened eardrum. Cotton swabs are also very irritating to a friable epithelium, and their use may result in painful abrasion or ulceration of the canal epithelium.

Only after the ear canal has been cleaned and dried can a determination of the integrity of the eardrum be made. Unfortunately, severely stenotic ear canals often prevent adequate visualization of the eardrum through the otoscope.

Examining the Ear Canal

For examination of the cleaned, dry ear canal, it is helpful to determine whether the otitis externa is acute or chronic. Chronic otitis externa is characterized by epithelial hyperkeratosis, glandular hyperplasia, fibrosis, stricture, and inflammatory cell infiltration of the dermis of the external auditory canal. The changes in surface contour of the ear canal caused by chronic otitis lead to formation of folds; routine flushing helps uncover offending organisms hidden deep in these folds so that topical antibiotics can gain access to the deeper epithelium.

Pathological changes associated with otitis externa may extend the entire length of the ear canal and may affect the tympanic membrane. One report involving histopathological evaluation of postmortem specimens from dogs with chronic otitis demonstrated that hair and keratin originating from the external ear were often found in the middle ear. The tympanic membrane in these specimens could not be identified histologically in a

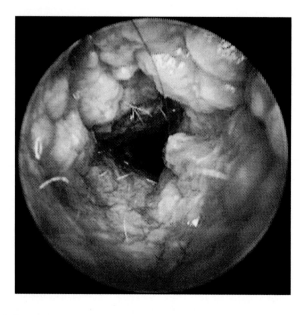

Figure 6–5

Chronic otitis externa is characterized by epithelial proliferation and fibrosis, resulting in an uneven epithelial surface contour. This photo was taken after the ear canal was flushed and dried.

significant number of cases, and when it could be identified, it was often thickened.

When the eardrum is ruptured, exudates drain from the external ear canal into the tympanic bulla. The mucous membrane lining the bulla, the *mucoperiosteum,* becomes inflamed and can produce copious exudate, which complicates the continued treatment of otitis externa (see Fig. 6–2). Liquid medications placed into the external ear canal cannot reach the bulla if the canal is already filled with mucus and pus.

Perpetuating Factors

Because of the changes in the ear canal that occur as a result of disease, bacteria and yeasts colonize and reproduce. Otitis externa is complicated by the growth of these infectious organisms, which is secondary to a primary disease process. Although antimicrobial therapy may temporarily relieve the symptoms of otitis externa, they may recur unless the underlying disease is identified and treated as well. Concomitant growth and colonization by these organisms are considered to be *perpetuating factors* in ear disease.

Colonizing organisms associated with otitis externa include bacteria and yeasts. Members of the genera *Malassezia, Staphylococcus,* and *Pseudomonas* are the organisms most commonly isolated from the ears of dogs. *Corynebacterium, Enterococcus,* and *Proteus* are also frequently isolated. The prevalence of one organism over another is determined by a variety of factors. For example, excessive cerumen production permits *Malassezia* growth, whereas the decreased immune function seen with hypothyroidism allows colonization by *Staphylococcus.*

Epidemiological reports from investigators around the world indicate a wide variety of prevalent organisms found in the ears of dogs with otitis externa. *Malassezia pachydermatis* is commonly found in the author's Alabama practice, but a report from Spain indicates that *Candida albicans* is the most prevalent otic fungal organism isolated there. Interpretation of the literature concerning the most prevalent organisms isolated from ear disease may therefore need to be regionalized. In addition, prevalent organisms may be determined by breed susceptibility to certain primary disease states that result in otitis. For example, acute otitis externa or otitis media in German shepherds frequently is perpetuated by a secondary *Pseudomonas* infection.

Isolates from the external ear canal do not always correlate with the isolates from the middle ear. *Pseudomonas* may be found more often in the middle ear than the external ear, whereas *Malassezia* is rarely found in the middle ear when the eardrum is intact. Some organisms rarely isolated from the external ear canal of dogs, such as β-hemolytic streptococci, may be found as the prevalent organism in otitis media.

Frequently, otitis externa resists topical treatment because infection extends through the tympanic membrane into the tympanic bulla, causing otitis media. This secondary otitis media occurs in approximately 16% of cases of acute otitis externa and in as many as 50% of cases of chronic otitis externa. Primary otitis media (extension of infection from the nasopharynx through the auditory tube to the tympanic bulla) is rare in the dog but is often seen in cats with nasopharyngeal polyps.

Studies in dogs have suggested that otitis media may be more common than previously recognized. In many dogs with otitis externa with intact eardrums, significant bacterial populations may also be isolated from the middle ear. These dogs may have had eardrum ruptures that healed, trapping bacteria in the tympanic bullae.

Treatment

Corticosteroids have a definite place in the treatment of otitis externa. Systemic corticosteroids reduce both the intense pruritus associated with acute otitis externa and the inflammation in the epithelium of the ear canal. Systemic corticosteroids are used for several days to reduce the edema and stenosis that prevent adequate examination of the ear canal. If the ear canal is patent, a potent topical corticosteroid, such as dexamethasone, betamethasone, or fluocinolone, may be used to relieve the intense pain and itching. As the otitis resolves, a less potent corticosteroid such as 1% hydrocortisone may be used in the ear to prevent inflammation in atopic dogs that may have recurrent otitis.

Antibiotics that kill *Staphylococcus, Pseudomonas,* and other gramnegative bacteria are used in many otic preparations. They may be formulated with other topical pharmaceuticals, such as antifungals, corticosteroids, insecticides, and topical anesthetics. Antibiotics such as gentamicin, neomycin, and polymyxin B are potentially ototoxic, so if the patient has no eardrum, these antibiotics should be avoided. In addition, neomycin has been implicated as a sensitizer in contact dermatitis in the ear. If the ear becomes worse with neomycin treatment, the antibiotic should be stopped immediately.

Although not labeled for otic use, injectable fluoroquinolone is used by the author in a variety of forms. It may be instilled directly into the ear as a bulla infusion to obtain very high tissue levels quickly. An enrofloxacin topical otic solution can be made by mixing 2 mL of injectable enrofloxacin with 13 mL of artificial tears. Also, 2 mL of injectable enrofloxacin (Baytril Injection, Bayer) mixed in an 8-mL bottle of dimethyl sulfoxide (DMSO) with fluocinolone (Synotic) provides a potent antibiotic, anti-inflammatory combination. This solution is unstable and should not be used for more than 5 days. Ciprofloxacin 0.3% eye drops can also be used in the ear. A new topical otic fluoroquinolone, ofloxacin, has been shown to be safe and effective in children with suppurative otitis media.

Ticarcillin has been used in severe cases of *Pseudomonas* otitis externa, both as a topical infusion into the tympanic bulla and as an intravenous antibiotic. This antibiotic is very expensive, and the intravenous route of administration requires the patient to be in the hospital for treatment. A treatment regimen is described using 1 to 2 mg/kg prednisolone per os once daily and a cleansing and drying ear cleaner, followed by topical administration of injectable ticarcillin solution four times daily. The patient with a ruptured eardrum receives 15 to 25 mg/kg ticarcillin three times daily intravenously until the membrane heals. Topical ticarcillin and the ear cleaner are continued twice daily for 14 days after clinical resolution. The duration of treatment ranges from 14 to 36 days. Reactions to intravenous ticarcillin have been seen in the dog.

Silver sulfadiazine cream has been used for treatment of resistant *Pseudomonas* infections. A small amount of the cream is dispersed in a volume of normal saline to make a 1% solution and is used as an ear drop twice daily. This compound has the potential to cause inflammation in the ear canal and may be ototoxic.

Another useful compound for resistant ear infections is ethylene-diamine tetraacetic acid–tris (EDTA-tris) solution. (TrizEDTA, DermaPet, Inc.) The solution can be mixed up in the veterinary hospital and dispensed fresh (see Box). EDTA-tris is particularly useful for otitis externa or otitis media caused by gram-negative bacteria. It affects the cell membranes of bacteria by chelating minerals such as calcium and magnesium, rendering the membranes more porous so that the antibiotic can diffuse into the bacteria and kill them. Even if culture and sensitivity results indicate that a gram-negative bacterium is resistant to a certain antibiotic in vitro, pretreatment with EDTA-tris may render the organism sensitive to the antibiotic in vivo. EDTA-tris is used as a pretreatment in the external ear 15 minutes prior to the instillation of topical antibiotics, most of which require an alkaline medium for maximum efficacy.

For otitis externa complicated by *Malassezia,* the author prefers the use of an acetic acid–boric acid solution (DermaPet Ear/Skin Cleaner).

EDTA-TRIS EAR SOLUTION FOR GRAM-NEGATIVE EAR INFECTIONS

How to Make

1. Mix:

EDTA (disodium salt)	1.2 g
Tris (tromethamine) (Trizma, Sigma Chemical)	6.05 g
Distilled water	1000 mL
Glacial acetic acid	1 mL

2. Adjust pH to 8.0 with additional glacial acetic acid.
3. Autoclave and store sterile.
4. Dispense in 4-oz bottles. Keep refrigerated.

How to Use (Twice Daily)

1. Fill ear canal with EDTA-tris solution.
2. Wait 15 minutes, and then wipe out any excess with a cotton ball.
3. Immediately instill antibiotic solution into the ear canal.

Alterations in cerumen lipid composition caused by underlying skin diseases such as atopy or hypothyroidism may play a role in the pathogenesis of *Malassezia* otitis externa. Low levels of free fatty acids in surface lipids coupled with increased levels of surface triglycerides favor *Malassezia* infections. The cleansing and desquamating effects of the acetic acid–boric acid solution essentially remove fatty acid substrates necessary for the metabolism and reproduction of *Malassezia*. This organism produces a chemotactic factor for neutrophils that is a hydrophilic protein. The presence of this factor may help explain why only a few *Malassezia* organisms can cause such profound erythema and pruritus. The cleansing effect of the acetic acid–boric acid solution removes this chemoattractant and may account for the reduction in inflammation. Boric acid, which is hygroscopic (drying out the humid ear canal), removes moisture necessary for this hydrophilic chemoattractant.

It has been demonstrated that more than 50% of atopic dogs with pruritic skin disease may have increased cutaneous *Malassezia* populations. Humans with atopic dermatitis also demonstrate *Malassezia* infections. With *Malassezia* otitis externa, treatment failures are frequent even though there appears to be temporary resolution of symptoms. Presumably, these "relapses" are often related to the initial diminution of inflammation due to the corticosteroid utilized in the ear medications or administered parenterally in atopic patients. The reduction in inflammation reduces clinical symptoms, but when the topical medication is discontinued and the infectious organism is still present, symptoms of erythema and pruritus reappear.

Follow-up

Because veterinarians rely on pet owners to follow their prescribed therapeutic protocols, time spent explaining proper ear care to clients helps them treat their animals' ears as prescribed. Clients should understand the need for frequent rechecks to monitor the progress of the pet with otitis externa. Too often, a patient is sent home with ear drops and then is not seen again until the otitis externa flares up. Scheduling a recheck visit allows the veterinarian to change therapy if there is no response.

The external canal can be cleaned by the owner at home to facilitate removal of excessive exudate accumulation associated with otitis externa or otitis media. The author prefers an acetic acid–boric acid solution for *Malassezia* infection and TrizEDTA (DermaPet, Inc.) for bacterial otitis for home use, because they are antiseptic and non-ototoxic. The procedure is as follows:

1. The ear canal is filled with the cleaning solution until it overflows.
2. The canal is externally massaged for 5 minutes.

3. The loosened debris is wiped off the external opening of the ear canal with a dry cotton ball.

This procedure is repeated daily at home until the recheck visit.

A good prognostic sign that uncomplicated otitis externa is resolving is to see regrowth of hair in the vertical canal. Most of the exudates formed in the acute phase of otitis externa have a depilatory effect on the hair follicle, so the hair falls out. When the inflammation subsides and the exudates are not dissolving hairs, hair regrowth can occur.

Frequently, after the otitis externa has resolved, the client is willing to allow the veterinarian to look for the underlying cause of the ear disease with a hypoallergenic food trial, allergy testing, or endocrine assays. Failure to identify and treat any underlying disease results in chronic otitis externa.

Suggested Readings

Foster AP, DeBoer DJ: The role of *Pseudomonas* in canine ear disease. Compend Cont Ed 20:909–918, 1998.

Gotthelf LN, Young SE: New treatment of *Malassezia* otitis externa in dogs. Vet Forum 14:46–53, 1997.

Harvey RG: Aspects of the interaction between skin and staphylococci. Bayer Selected Proceedings of the North American Veterinary Conference, January 1998, pp 79–84.

Kiss G, Radvanyi S, Szigeti G: New combination for the therapy of canine otitis externa: Microbiology of otitis externa and efficacy in vivo and in vitro. J Small Anim Pract 38:51–60, 1997.

Merchant SR, Bellah JJ: Otitis Symposium. Vet Med 92:517–550, 1997.

Nuttall TJ: Use of ticarcillin in the management of canine otitis externa complicated by *Pseudomonas aeruginosa*. J Small Anim Pract 39:165–168, 1998.

Powell MB, Weisbroth SH, Roth L, Wilhelmsen C: Reaginic hypersensitivity in *Otodectes cyanotis* infestation of cats and mode of mite feeding. Am J Vet Res 41:877–882, 1980.

Trevor PB, Martin RA: Tympanic bulla osteotomy for treatment of middle-ear disease in cats: 19 cases (1984–1991). J Am Vet Med Assoc 202:123–128, 1993.

7

Allergic
Otitis Externa

Michael Groh, DVM

In the John August classification of primary, predisposing, and perpetuating causes of otitis externa, allergy is one of the primary causes, and probably the most common. If unrecognized, mismanaged or ignored, allergy in most cases leads to bacterial or yeast infection or both, which are the leading causes of chronic otic disease. It is then usually only a matter of time before chronic otitis externa leads to pyoderma or *Malassezia* dermatitis, thus confounding the recognition of underlying allergy. It is important for the clinician to maintain a high index of suspicion for the presence of allergy and to resist the temptation to employ corticosteroids in the early treatment of otitis.

A case can be made for the use of systemic or topical steroids for otitis externa (1) in advanced disease that threatens to become irreversible or (2) when pain and swelling must be managed. Steroids are also indicated in end-stage disease when owners decline further therapy. Because all commercially available topical otic preparations currently contain steroids of varying potency, however, the clinician must compound his or her own topical preparations if steroids are to be avoided. These compounded preparations are selected according to results of otic cytological evaluation and include 0.5% or 1% silver sulfadiazine, miconazole lotion, and clotrimazole solution for yeast infection. If cytological evaluation reveals cocci or bacilli, injectable enrofloxacin may be added to silver sulfadiazine for an elegant broad-spectrum topical preparation. Other suggestions for mixed infections are gentamicin and amikacin mixed with silver sulfadiazine or clotrimazole.

Ototoxicity is always a concern with topical therapy, but so is uncontrolled infection. Systemic antibiotics should always be prescribed concurrently with topical therapy when a dermatitis is present or if the tympanic membrane appears discolored, thickened, or perforated. Systemic antibiotics are also selected according to results of otic cytological evaluation and may be combined when necessary into a polypharmacy approach—for example, silver sulfadiazine with enrofloxacin in a topical preparation or ketoconazole and cephalexin for oral administration. In these cases, the patient should be rechecked frequently with cytological evaluations and otic lavage until the infection is resolved. If the pruritus also resolves with this steroid-free approach, allergy can usually be ruled out.

An exception might be food allergy, which is capable of producing recurring or persistent otitis and pyoderma. If allergy is ruled out, a cursory search for other underlying diseases should be considered at the very least. If potential allergic symptoms persist despite steroid-free infection control, however, they may then be aggressively pursued.

Allergic Otitis

The precise mechanisms of allergy are not well understood, but it appears that allergy in small animal medicine results from either an antibody-mediated (immediate-type) hypersensitivity, as in atopy, or a cell-mediated (delayed-type) hypersensitivity, as in contact allergy (or cutaneous drug eruption). Both types of hypersensitivity may result in otitis externa, and although other hypersensitivity reactions may play a role, the scope of this chapter is limited to discussion of immediate and delayed allergies.

Immediate hypersensitivity is responsible for the clinical symptoms of aeroallergy and probably plays a role in food allergy and hormonal hypersensitivity. Delayed hypersensitivity is responsible for topical drug reactions and, although the issue is controversial, may be involved in some food allergy reactions.

Immediate Hypersensitivity (Atopy)

Atopy is an antibody-mediated, adverse inflammatory reaction mounted by a genetically predisposed individual against an antigenic substance to which a non-predisposed individual would be nonreactive. An antigen capable of sensitizing an individual becomes an *allergen*. Factors influencing the development of atopy, besides genetic predisposition, may be the timing of first allergen exposure and, at least in humans, the concentration and size of the initial sensitizing allergen.

Exposure to allergen occurs via inhalation and probably ingestion (aeroallergens and foods), but percutaneous absorption may be the major route of exposure for aeroallergens. The immune mechanisms associated with atopy are poorly understood. Allergens are presented to antibody-producing cells by helper T cells in the dermis or submucosa and by dendritic cells within the epidermis.

Allergen-specific immunoglobulin E (IgE), and probably IgG (IgGd subclass) are subsequently produced and, via the circulatory system, adhere to receptor sites on mast cells in the skin. Upon re-exposure of the individual to specific allergen, mast cell degranulation occurs, releasing pharmacologically active inflammatory mediators that produce the pruritic clinical symptoms of atopic dermatitis.

Aeroallergy

Aeroallergy, as a form of atopy, derives its name from airborne particles that are capable of becoming allergens. Important aeroallergens in dogs and cats are dust particles (house dust and, to some extent, grain dusts), pollens, molds, and insect or arachnid fecal allergens and decomposing body parts. Included in this last group are the ubiquitous house dust mites. Aeroallergens may have a definite seasonality, depending on the geographical location and the involved allergen. Humid tropical and subtropical climates may produce nonseasonal insect, arachnid, and mold allergens. Of lesser importance, animal danders may be nonseasonal in any environment.

Aeroallergy has been estimated to be the second most common canine allergy, flea allergy dermatitis being the first. With the greater efficacy of the new-generation ovicides and topical adulticides, however, the incidence of flea allergy is dropping. Of confirmed cases of aeroallergy, otitis may occur in half, although otitis as the only sign of atopy remains uncommon. When present, it usually involves the concave surface of the pinna and the skin contiguous with the opening of the ear canal more than the ear canal proper. It is tempting to postulate that canal cerumen reduces the percutaneous component of the disease, thereby lessening the reaction within the canal. An additional sign of aeroallergy is pruritus of the face, feet, ventrum, perineum, or tailhead. Erythema may or may not be present.

Diagnosis

Diagnosis of aeroallergy can be confirmed via intradermal skin tests, when performed by an experienced clinician using fresh, properly diluted antigens. In most cases, intradermal skin tests are not cost-effective for the average clinician performing few tests. Results of the in vitro enzyme-linked immunosorbent assays (ELISAs) now available do not correlate well with skin test results, although immunotherapy based on in vitro tests, in some meticulously chosen patients, has been shown to achieve improvement similar to that of conventional, skin test–based immunotherapy.

Success with either method requires careful interpretation of the results. The clinician must ensure that any positive results correlate well with the patient history, because the sole purpose of specific diagnosis of aeroallergy is to guide in the selection of treatment antigens. Poorly chosen treatment antigens yield poor immunotherapy results. In addition, successful immunotherapy also requires frequent consultations to manage the day-to-day variation in clinical signs brought about by fluctuations in aeroallergen concentrations and close monitoring of the advancing immunotherapy dosages.

In its uncomplicated state, in the absence of infection and concurrent disease, aeroallergy is responsive to steroids at relatively low therapeutic doses and, in some cases, may respond in part to antihistamines or essential fatty acids. Avoidance therapies, such as remaining in air conditioning, frequent bathing, and regular wiping of the face and paws after coming indoors, may also be helpful in reducing allergen exposure to varying degrees.

Food Allergy

The immunological mechanisms of food allergy are unknown. Because ingestion of allergenic foods in the genetically predisposed individual often results in clinical symptoms within minutes or hours, immediate hypersensitivity is clearly present.

Examples of some common immediate reactions are panting, polydipsia, urticaria, angioedema, behavior changes, erythema, and, occasionally, pruritus. When erythema and pruritus are present, they often involve the ear. Whether IgE, IgG, or both are involved in these reactions remains unresolved.

A non-IgE, or modified IgE, reaction is supported by the fact that results of IgE-based, in vitro ELISAs and intradermal skin tests are discordant with results of single-food provocative exposure trials. One must consider, however, that the food extracts used in these tests are not standardized and may also contribute to the discordant results. Some reactions in food-allergic patients also appear to have a delayed onset ranging from a few hours to days. One must be careful to ensure that so-called delayed food allergy reactions are not, in fact, late-phase bacterial or yeast infections. These disorders may be manifested clinically on the skin surface and within the ear canal and can be documented cytologically. As previously mentioned, systemic antibiotics are preferred over systemic steroids when infectious organisms are found.

Also, some cases of delayed-onset dermatitis and otitis, particularly in provocative exposure feeding trials, may be mistaken for delayed hypersensitivity reactions. This phenomenon is not fully understood, but could be explained by high tolerance to pruritogenic mast cell substances, reduced number of activated mast cells, or, simply, mild food allergy. In any case, these altered states of atopic food allergy dermatitis can be misdiagnosed as delayed food allergy.

Diagnosis

At present, neither intradermal skin tests nor in vitro ELISAs are accurate in diagnosing food allergy. Each has better negative than positive predictive values, and results of both are discordant with those of food elimination and subsequent provocative exposure. It has also been inaccurately suggested that food allergy is refractory to steroid therapy and therefore easily distinguished from aeroallergy. In reality, a significant percentage of uncomplicated food allergies actually respond well to steroids. Food exclusion trials using novel home-cooked foods or sufficiently hydrolyzed commercial diets, such as EXclude and Veterinary Exclusion Diet, are currently the only reliable and reproducible methods of diagnosis. As in testing for aeroallergy, steroid-free infection control should be employed and parasites must be controlled or ruled out prior to or concurrently with food exclusion.

Once food allergy is confirmed, single-food provocation or trial-and-error testing with home-cooked or commercial diets may be used to determine a suitable maintenance diet. This phase can be frustrating for both clinician and client, especially when an animal has multiple food allergies. Because no universally hypoallergenic diet is commercially available at this time, some difficult cases may require maintenance with systemic antibiotics.

Hormonal Hypersensitivity

The immunology of hormonal hypersensitivity, a rare canine disease, is poorly understood, but immediate and delayed skin test reactions to endogenous sex hormones have been demonstrated. Most cases have been reported in intact females and begin as a pruritic, erythematous, or papulocrustous dermatitis involving the tailhead, perineum, genital and ventral abdomen, or caudomedial thighs. Advanced cases can involve the face and ears, producing an inflammatory disease nearly indistinguishable from food allergy or severe aeroallergy.

As with other types of allergic disease, a high index of suspicion and a steroid-free evaluation are prerequisites for an accurate and timely diagnosis. History is also important in diagnosing these cases, because early in the disease, most females demonstrate the dermatitis only during estrous or, to a lesser extent, false pregnancy. In later stages, the disease in females resembles the naturally occurring nonseasonal disease of males.

Definitive diagnosis is usually made from the response to ovariohysterectomy or castration, when permitted. The infectious otitis component of the disease, as in other allergies, is managed with the rational use of topical and systemic antibiotics guided by results of cytological evaluation.

Allergic Contact Dermatitis (Cutaneous Drug Eruption)

A rarely reported disease, allergic contact dermatitis occurs as a result of type IV, delayed hypersensitivity reaction due to repeated topical exposure to an allergenic substance. The disease is pruritic and produces erythema, edema, eruptions of papular crusts, and ulceration. It usually occurs only in sparsely haired areas and in the ear.

Naturally occurring disease results from exposure to a relatively short list of plant varieties or extracts and a more extensive list of manufactured allergens. The list of these types of allergens is outside the scope of this discussion, because the major causes of otic contact allergy are the topical agents used in managing otitis. Neomycin has long been recognized as a cause of allergic contact dermatitis in humans, which occurs rarely in veterinary medicine as well. Other substances shown to be contact allergens are silver sulfadiazine, cleansers, topical anesthetics, insecticides, and tars.

Diagnosis is made through recognition that the otitis either worsens in conjunction with use of the agent or "fails to respond" to rational use of appropriate therapies. Definitive diagnosis is made upon documentation of improvement after withdrawal of and exacerbation following provocative exposure to the suspected topical agent.

8

Otitis Media

Louis N. Gotthelf, DVM

A common sequela of external ear disease in dogs is destruction of the eardrum, which gives foreign material and infectious organisms access to the respiratory tissues lining the middle ear. The reaction of these mucous membranes is different from the reaction of the skin of the external ear, so the symptomatology and treatment of otitis media are different from those of otitis externa.

Patients with otitis media have a history of chronic or recurrent ear infections. Almost all of them have otorrhea, which causes the sensation of liquid in the ears, and they shake their heads to relieve the abnormal sensation. Patients in which otitis media is suspected are presented for ear treatment after having been previously treated topically for otitis externa. Their ear disease no longer responds to the topical therapy. Otoscopic examination reveals liquid exudate filling the ear canal. Middle ear tumors or polyps may be present under the liquid. Sometimes, the overflow of the exudate collects on the hair at the pinnal entrance to the ear canal. Middle ear disease may lead to a hearing deficit or a vestibular dysfunction. Head tilt, ataxia, and circling may result. In addition, behavioral changes due to the severe pain of otitis media may be evident.

Signalment and History

Acute otitis media is rarely found in the dog and cat. It is uncommon for a patient to present to the veterinarian with acute otitis media. More commonly, a dog with otitis media will have the history of recurrent or chronic ear infections. Perhaps the pet owner will bring in all the ear medications already tried on the pet; that is a signal for the veterinarian to look deeper in the ear canal for middle ear disease.

Dogs and cats with otitis media often have a liquid discharge present when the ear canal is examined with the otoscope. Some patients will produce so much exudate that it will overflow onto the periaural region of the face, or in a floppy-eared dog, there will be dried exudate on the ear flap adjacent to the external opening of the auditory canal. Head shaking to relieve the tickle associated with liquid exudate is very common in otitis media. Pain on palpation of the base of the ear canal or pain on manipulation of the pinna should also alert the clinician to otitis media. Some patients with otitis media are reluctant to have the mouth opened, and there may be a history of reluctance to chew hard food. This is due to inflammation and swelling within the bulla, which is located adjacent to the temporomandibular joint.

When otitis media affects the nerves that course through the tympanic bullae, the patient may show signs as subtle as keratoconjunctivitis sicca on the ipsilateral side. Sometimes there are mild signs of Horner's syndrome (enophthalmos, ptosis, and miosis). Some patients may show pain, head tilt, or a drooped lip, drooped ear, or loss of the ability to close the eyelid leading to exposure keratitis. Peripheral vestibular disease with nystagmus and circling may be evident if the infection and inflammation have affected the inner ear.

Some owners will present the dog for a hearing deficit. Fluid in the middle ear dampens acute hearing. When the eardrum is ruptured or when the ossicles of the middle ear have sclerosed, air conduction hearing is reduced. High-pitched sound waves cannot be effectively transmitted from the ear canal to the cochlea. If a tumor or a polyp has filled the middle ear, air conduction hearing is eliminated. Bone conduction hearing is usually still present in these patients, and the pet can hear only the lower range of tones. (Bone conduction hearing can be demonstrated by placing your fingers in your ears and listening to the sounds around you.)

If there is pharyngeal drainage of mucus and exudates, the patient may be presented for stridor. In these cases, a pharyngeal examination may reveal a nasopharyngeal polyp interfering with breathing or thick mucus covering the caudal pharynx and occluding the airway.

Otitis media in dogs and cats is much more prevalent than previously thought. Many cases are well hidden from visual detection because of the severe pathological changes that have occurred in the ear canal as a result of chronic otitis externa. Stenosis, fibrosis, tumors, and epithelial hyperplasia prevent adequate visualization beyond these blockages, so determining the integrity of the eardrum is not always possible (Fig. 8–1). Healed eardrums trap infectious organisms in the middle ear, and otitis media without communication to the external canal often results; examination in such cases shows an intact eardrum (Fig. 8–2). However, the eardrum may change color in response to inflammation on the medial side. Frequently, the tympanic membrane will become very opaque and gray in color, rather than pearly and translucent. Sometimes there is fluid behind the eardrum and examination of the intact tympanic membrane may indicate that it is bulging into the external ear. Purulent material in the middle ear may be seen as yellow fluid behind the eardrum. Early polyps and tumors in the middle ear may be seen as fleshy masses through the eardrum.

Evaluating the Eardrum

When the eardrum cannot be seen otoscopically, proper patient preparation facilitates the examination. Systemic or topical corticosteroids may be given for a few days to reduce inflammation and increase lumen diameter. Chemical restraint or anesthesia may be required just to examine a fractious dog with a suspected ruptured eardrum. When otitis media is complicated by a liquid exudate or caseated material, gentle flushing of

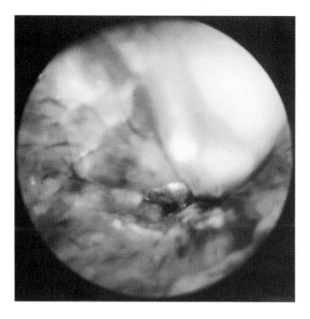

Figure 8–1

Assessment of the integrity of the eardrum is difficult if not impossible in a stenotic ear.

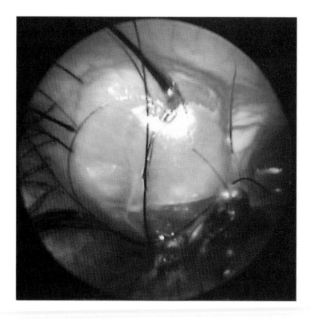

Figure 8–2

After the eardrum heals, otitis media may still be present. This healed eardrum is bulging from fluid pressure behind it in the tympanic bulla.

the external ear canal is indicated. Otitis media is a very painful disease process, so topical or parenteral anesthetics may be used to decrease pain.

Determining the Integrity of the Eardrum

Several techniques have been described to determine the integrity of the tympanic membrane. A small rigid catheter or a Spreull needle can be inserted into the ear canal until it stops. It is then extended and retracted to get a feel for the rigidity of the "stop." If there is a spongy feel, the eardrum is intact. If there is a definite hard feel to the "stop," the eardrum is ruptured and the catheter is hitting the medial wall of the tympanic bulla.

Pressure tympanometry can be performed by inserting a bulb syringe filled with air into the ear canal to seal off the external ear canal. The air is gently squeezed into the ear, and if air comes out of the auditory tube in the pharynx, the eardrum is ruptured. The author prefers to use a warmed dilute povidone iodine solution for this technique. If the orange flushing fluid comes out of the nose or out through the oropharynx, the eardrum is ruptured.

Another technique used by some is to fill the ear canal with warmed saline and to insert the tip of a video otoscope (Video Vetscope, MedRx, Inc., Seminole, FL) into the ear canal. By looking through the clear fluid, if air bubbles rise from the eardrum while the animal breathes, then the eardrum is ruptured, allowing air from the nasopharynx to escape from the middle ear. The rising bubbles indicate a ruptured eardrum.

Positive contrast radiography has been described as a method for detecting a ruptured tympanic membrane in dogs with otitis media. Two to five ml of dilute iodinated contrast agent was instilled into the normal ear canals of cadavers with intact eardrums that were intentionally ruptured. In every case, contrast media entered the tympanic bulla and was detected by radiography. In clinical otitis media cases, canalography was positive in most of the cases in which the eardrum was determined to be ruptured otoscopically and was positive in other cases in which the eardrum appeared to be intact otoscopically. In normal ears, canalography was more accurate for detecting iatrogenic TM perforation than otoscopy.

Anatomy of the Tympanic Membrane and Tympanic Bulla

A review of the histology of the tympanic membrane is needed to explain the events leading to otitis media. The tympanic membrane in the dog is a thin, translucent structure composed of three layers. The outer layer, in the external ear canal, consists of germinal epithelium one or two cells thick. The next is the middle collagen layer to which the epithelium is attached; there are radial and circular collagen fibers in this thin supporting structure (Fig. 8–3). The innermost or third layer is composed of a single layer of flat, squamous epithelium that is continuous with the cuboidal epithelium lining the tympanic bulla and covering the auditory ossicles.

The tympanic cavity is a hollow spherical bony structure of the petrous temporal bone medial to the eardrum. Dorsally, it contains the auditory ossicles, the chorda tympani nerve coursing just behind the dorsal aspect of the malleus bone, and the round and oval windows to the internal ear (see Chapter 1). The auditory tube connecting the middle ear with the nasopharynx is located on the medial dorsal wall. In this area lie the sympathetic nerves and ganglia associated with branches of the facial and trigeminal nerves. The remaining ventral portion, or fundus, is the tympanic bulla, an air-filled cuplike structure of bone. The diameter of the tympanic bulla is approximately three to four times that of the external ear canal, so the bulla is capable of containing a large volume of fluid. It is lined by a thin layer of cuboidal epithelium that is continuous with the columnar epithelium of the auditory tube.

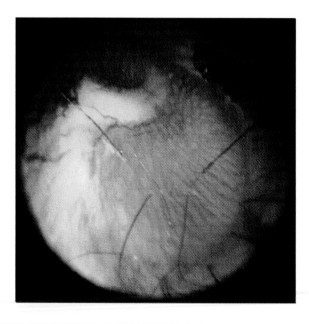

Figure 8–3

Normal canine eardrum reveals radiating collagen fibers forming the pars tensa.

Pathogenesis

Tissue reactions in the external ear canal vary according to the causative organism, the character of the inflammatory exudates, the enzymes elaborated, the diameter of the horizontal and vertical canals, and the effects of other underlying skin diseases, such as atopy, hypothyroidism, and seborrheic disease.

Exudates and organisms draining into the middle ear through an eroded or ruptured eardrum get trapped in the ventral portion of the bulla. (Samples for cytological evaluation or culture should be taken from the ventral bulla prior to suctioning.) The resulting suppurative inflammation causes the lining epithelium in the bulla to change from cuboidal to pseudostratified columnar, leading to an increase in the number of secretory cells and glands, which add to the quantity of exudate.

The lamina propria thickens in response to inflammation, and as vascularity increases, edema and granulation tissue result. As otitis media becomes more chronic, the lamina propria changes to dense connective tissue, and bone spicules may develop within it.

"False Middle Ear" and Cholesteatoma

Obstructions along the horizontal ear canal from hypertrophic glands, neoplasia, inflammation, or ceruminous plugs increase pressure on the tympanic membrane, causing it to bulge into the middle ear cavity. Coupled with poor air movement through the eustachian tube, negative pressure inside the bulla pulls the eardrum even farther into the middle ear cavity. A "false middle ear" may develop when the distended membrane balloons into the bulla and may be misdiagnosed as a ruptured eardrum.

The invaginating eardrum may collect large amounts of debris from the external canal, such as keratin, wax, and desquamated epithelial cells. *Cholesteatoma,* a rare inflammatory condition of the middle ear in dogs and cats, results in thickening and abnormal growth of the invaginated tympanic membrane epithelium into the middle ear cavity. Cholesteatoma may be congenital (Fig. 8–4) or may result from otitis media.

In acquired cholesteatoma, hyperproliferative squamous epithelium from the mucocutaneous junctions grows into the middle ear cavity in an uncontrolled manner. After perforation of the tympanic membrane or epidermal injury, the migrating keratinocytes at the leading edge of the damaged epithelium fail to cover the perforation. Instead, they grow toward the medial side of the eardrum. Bacterial infection at the site of the perforation seems to accelerate the proliferation of keratinocytes

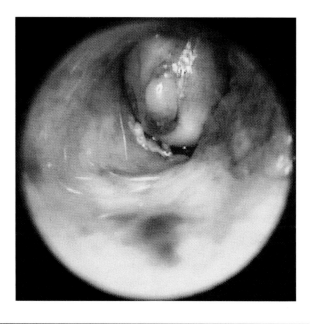

Figure 8-4

Congenital cholesteatoma in a cat. The epithelial cyst was ruptured at surgery, revealing a thick secretion contained in a saclike structure.

under the influence of cytokines, especially interleukin-1α. Free keratin at the margin of the perforation causes intense inflammation at the mucocutaneous junction. During the body's attempt to heal the hole in the eardrum, the migrating hyperproliferative keratinized epithelium forms a pouch or cystic structure containing a core of keratin layers and inflammatory cells enclosed by the tympanic membrane.

Cholesteatoma seems to grow uncontrolled, almost like a tumor mass, enlarging with keratin and inflammatory cells. The large epidermal cyst may crowd out normal middle ear structures, including nerves and the auditory ossicles. When the pathogenesis of cholesteatoma was studied in rats, a hole in the pars flaccida was more likely to initiate cholesteatoma formation than a perforation of the pars tensa. The medial surface of the expanding cyst lies on the inflamed fibrous stroma within the middle ear and becomes attached to it, forming adhesions. Surgical removal of cholesteatoma from the tympanic bulla through a bulla osteotomy is required.

Cholesteatoma has a higher incidence in humans than in dogs or cats, for unknown reasons. Otitis media in humans usually results from infections of the throat that migrate into the middle ear through the eustachian tube. This type of infection seems to promote hyperproliferation of migrating keratinocytes when the eardrum perforates. In contrast, most middle ear infections in the dog and cat are secondary; an infection of the skin of the external ear extends through a tympanic membrane perforation into the middle ear. The resulting milieu may not contain the required stimulus for epithelial hyperproliferation.

Tympanic Membrane Rupture

Owing to the L configuration of the ear canal, proteolytic enzymes within exudates produced by otitis externa accumulate against the eardrum. The resulting inflammation and enzymatic destruction lead to necrosis of the epithelium and supporting collagen; thinning of the tympanic membrane causes it to weaken (Fig. 8–5). A healthy tympanic membrane can withstand pressures up to 300 mm Hg before it becomes damaged. The cytological architecture of an eardrum in an infected ear is sufficiently disrupted that it can withstand pressure of only 80 mm Hg before rupturing.

Ulceration along the ear canal can extend to the eardrum (Fig. 8–6). The ulcerated tissue leaks serum, which can cause maceration and exco-

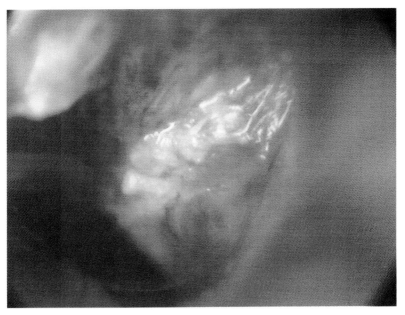

Figure 8–5

In otitis externa, exudates macerate the thin epithelial lining of the tympanic membrane. This close-up view of an eardrum reveals a thin, unhealthy appearance prior to impending rupture.

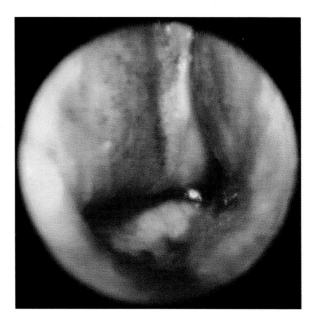

Figure 8–6

With ear canal ulceration from severe otitis externa, serum proteins come in contact with the ear canal epithelium, including the eardrum. This exposure results in erosion of the epithelium of the eardrum and can lead to rupture.

riation of the epithelium. The reaction is similar to a "hot spot" on the skin of the trunk of the dog. Liberation of bacterial proteases, release of lysozymes from phagocytic cells, and the epidermal maceration resulting from the excessive amount of serum in the ear canal disrupt the epithelial layers of the canal, either eroding or rupturing the eardrum.

Many cases of acute otitis media can be prevented. Special care in cleaning and flushing the external ear canal can prevent the high pressure from causing an iatrogenic rupture. Removal of exudates by careful flushing of the ear canal eliminates the source of destructive enzymes acting on the eardrum. Specific therapy for infectious organisms based on cytological or culture results can shorten the course of the bacterial or fungal disease. Treatment of underlying skin disease, such as atopy, food allergy, and hypothyroidism, may remove or control conditions that are primary causes of otitis externa. Proper client education concerning the chronic nature of ear diseases improves owner compliance by encouraging frequent rechecks to follow the progress of treatment. Recheck visits allow the veterinarian to make changes in the treatment protocol if response to therapy is inadequate.

Ototoxicity

The aminoglycosides, detergents, and most disinfectants routinely used in the treatment of the external ear canal are toxic to the nervous structures of the inner ear. When the eardrum is perforated or totally absent, these medications can gain access to the inner ear via the round and oval windows of the middle ear, resulting in neurological ototoxicity. Potentially ototoxic compounds are present in most topical formulations for treatment of otitis externa. Many ear-cleaning solutions contain a mixture of potentially ototoxic substances that may gain access to the inner ear and alter vestibular and cochlear function. Careful consideration of the ingredients contained in an ear cleaner is essential prior to its use. Many manufacturers are now indicating on the labels of such products that they should not be used if the eardrum is not intact (see Chapter 9).

The clinician should assess the risks of the topical use of a potentially ototoxic drug or ear flush solution versus its therapeutic benefits in the treatment of otitis media. The thin membranes of the round and oval windows in acute otitis media provide easier access into the inner ear for many of these compounds than the thickened membranes found in chronic otitis media. The round window, also known as a secondary tympanic membrane, may be affected by exudates contained within the tympanic bulla and may also become damaged. Access of ototoxins to the inner ear structures may be enhanced by damage to the round window.

Ototoxicity results from damage to either the cochlea or the vestibular apparatus. Gentamicin, for example, concentrates in the hair cells of the vestibular apparatus when administered parenterally. The cell permeability is altered so the hair cells swell and become deformed. They are rendered rigid and are unable to respond to movements of the endolymph. Ataxia, head tilt, and circling can result. A similar situation occurs in the cochlea when neomycin or kanamycin concentrates there. The cochlear nerve cells are damaged and cannot respond to vibrations, leading to hearing loss.

Radiographic Evaluation

Radiographic assessment of the bullae can be very helpful in determining the extent of bony involvement in otitis media. The absence of radiographic changes in the bulla does not rule out otitis media, however, especially in a recent case, because bony changes may not have had time to occur.

The first radiograph is an open-mouth, rostrocaudal view taken with the x-ray beam directed through the pharynx. The tongue should be pulled rostrally to remove soft tissue that overlies the bullae. Additional films can be obtained, including lateral oblique views of each bulla with the x-ray beam directed through the ramus of the mandible.

In a dog with minimal bony changes, the normal bullae appear as thin-walled circular structures medial to the mandibular rami on the rostro-caudal view. The cortical outline is thin, and the middle of each bulla is radiolucent because the bullae are filled with air. The cat has a two-chambered tympanic bulla separated by a bony septum (Fig. 8–7). When the bulla is affected by chronic disease, either the intraluminal or the extraluminal bone shows new bone production or remodeling (Fig. 8–8). The cartilage of the external canal may have also calcified and may be easily seen on a radiograph (Fig. 8–9). Often, an entire bulla appears radiopaque because large volumes of thick exudate or tissue growths fill the air space (Fig. 8–10). One or both bullae may be affected. If large volumes of flushing solution are infused into the ear canal of a dog with a ruptured eardrum prior to radiographic assessment, the radiograph can be misread, because the bulla filled with the flushing fluid appears radiopaque. One limitation of radiographic evaluation is that old sclerotic lesions in the bulla of an aged animal cannot be differentiated from a more current lesion from proliferative otitis media.

Computed tomography (CT) scanning of the tympanic bullae, if available, may aid in differentiating bony lesions in the bulla from soft tissue reactions. Even when the ear canal is stenotic and otoscopic examination is impossible, CT scans are able to give a clear impression of the status of the ear canal distal to the stenosis as well as clues to the disease in the middle ear. Bony lesions of the bulla can be differentiated from soft tissue lesions on CT scans (see Chapter 13).

Treatment

The clinician must consider several factors when planning therapy for otitis media:

1. The copious exudates produced and contained in the bulla must be removed, or they will overflow back into the external ear canal. When the fluid spills over into the horizontal canal, more inflammation, excoriation, and ulceration of the epidermis of the external canal result, inhibiting healing of the tympanic membrane (Fig. 8–11).

2. The inflammation in the bulla must be controlled with topical corticosteroids, systemic corticosteroids, or both.

3. Infectious organisms sequestered in deep crypts of the hyperplastic epithelial folds of the external ear canal, in sclerotic tissue of the submucosal layer, and in the crypts of the mucoperiosteum of the middle ear must be controlled with systemic antibiotic or antifungal agents.

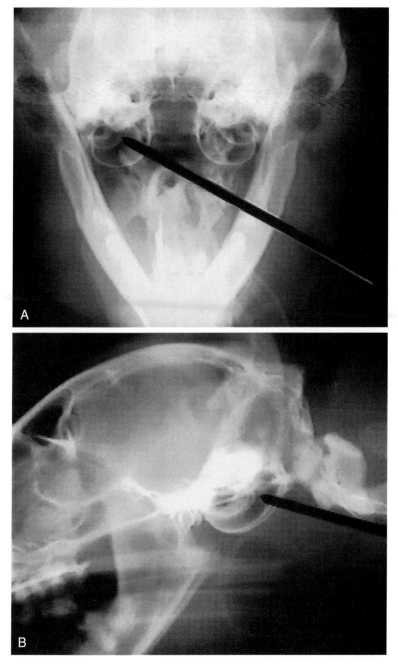

Figure 8–7

The double-walled tympanic bullae in the normal cat. *A*, Rostro-occipital open-mouth view. *B*, Lateral view. (*A* and *B* courtesy of Dr. Gary Lantz, Purdue University.)

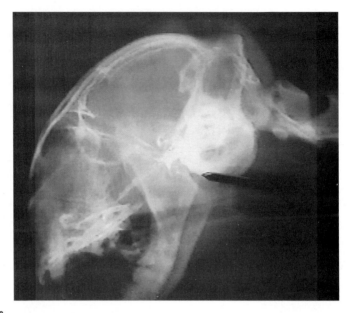

Figure 8–8

Lateral radiograph of a cat with severe otitis media and nasopharyngeal polyp. (Courtesy of Dr. Gary Lantz, Purdue University.)

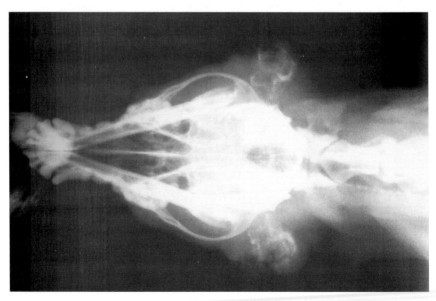

Figure 8–9

Dorsoventral radiograph of a 13-year-old Cocker spaniel with chronically calcified ear canals. Notice the ossification of the ear cartilage of both ear canals.

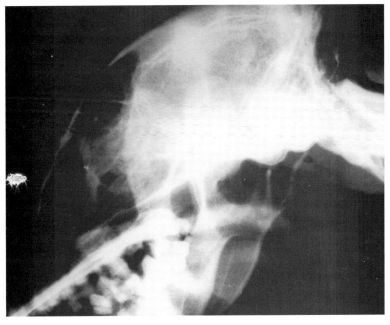

Figure 8–10

The tympanic bullae of a 9-year-old collie are completely filled with an iodine flushing solution. The thin bone of the bulla can be seen, indicating that the opacity is intraluminal and is not affecting the bone of the bulla.

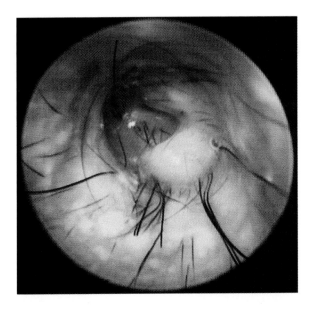

Figure 8–11

Otitis media in a young Labrador retriever. No eardrum was present in this dog, and hairs were found in the middle ear. Copious mucus and pus from a foreign body reaction fills the horizontal ear canal.

Flushing of the Tympanic Bulla

Once the diagnosis of otitis media is confirmed (Figs. 8–12 and 8–13), warmed saline or very dilute povidone-iodine solution is infused directly into the tympanic bulla. The flush solution is ejected under low pressure with a syringe and a red rubber urethral catheter or feeding tube cut to the proper length to extend into the bulla. Suctioning can be done with the same syringe and catheter or with the catheter connected to suction (Fig. 8–14). The catheter tip should always be directed ventrally to avoid the auditory ossicles and chorda tympani nerve, which are located dorsally.

A video otoscope (Video Vetscope, MedRx, Inc., Seminole, FL) makes suctioning of the tympanic bulla a simple, efficient procedure. A 5.5-inch open-ended tomcat catheter connected to suction is placed into the 2-mm working channel built into the video otoscope. The veterinarian positions the video otoscope in the proper location, and the assistant manipulates the catheter under direction from the veterinarian. The entire cleaning process is observed on the video monitor. Use of a suction pump allows small pieces of wax, mucus, pus, blood clots, and other material in the bulla to be removed quite easily without the need for an assistant to manipulate a suction syringe. Ear curettes can be used in the bulla to loosen

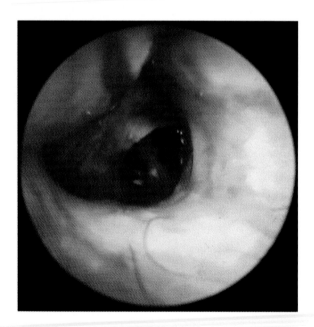

Figure 8–12

After the ear of a German shepherd was cleaned, a partial tear of the eardrum was revealed, confirming otitis media.

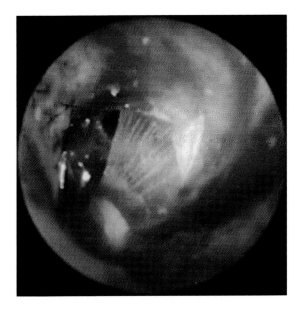

Figure 8–13

While the ears of a 8-year-old German shepherd with chronic ear disease were being flushed, the flush solution was seen draining out of the mouth. Examination revealed chronic otitis media. In otitis media, if the eustachian tube is patent, the flush solution can flow into the throat and nasopharynx.

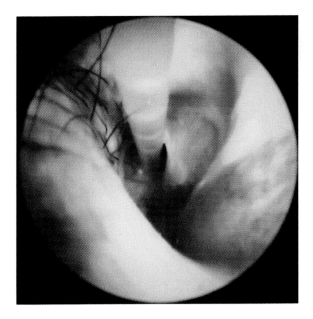

Figure 8–14

It is imperative that the middle ear be suctioned to remove debris that has accumulated in the bulla. This 5-year-old poodle has a persistent perforation of the eardrum, and its middle ear must be cleaned periodically.

firmly adherent material seen there. Curettes can puncture through the bulla if there is any lysis of the eggshell-thin bone.

The flushing procedure is repeated until the bulla has been flushed and meticulously vacuumed to remove all foreign material. The white surface of the tympanic bulla can be seen through the otoscope when the bulla is clean. The entire bulla cannot be seen through an otoscope; only its medial wall can be visualized (Fig. 8–15). Often during this vacuuming procedure, disruption of the inflamed epithelium in the bulla causes bleeding.

Many nerves course through foramina in the petrous temporal bone and around the ear canal, including branches of the facial nerve and the trigeminal nerve. After flushing and suctioning of the middle ear, mechanical trauma from the instrumentation can affect nerve function. Some patients may show signs of pain, head tilt, Horner's syndrome (enophthalmos, ptosis, and miosis), drooped lip, drooped ear, or loss of the ability to close the eyelid. Although many of these clinical signs are transient, some patients may have irreversible damage. Some patients also show vestibular signs caused by iatrogenic extension of the infection to the inner ear and subsequently into the brain stem. Partial deafness can result even if the eardrum heals normally.

Repeated flushing of the tympanic bulla is usually required in patients with otitis media until the suppuration is reduced and the ear canal and

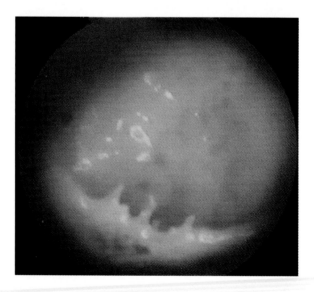

Figure 8–15

The sclerotic medial wall of the tympanic bulla can be seen in this close-up view. Note the irregular contour of the mucoperiosteum.

bulla remain dry. The owner needs to understand that the pet will be examined on a weekly basis with anesthesia and middle ear flushing until control of the infection is achieved.

Reduction of Inflammation

Once the tympanic cavity has been cleaned and dried, a topical corticosteroid, such as dimethyl sulfoxide (DMSO) with fluocinolone (Synotic, Syntex, Ft. Dodge, IA), is infused through a catheter placed into the bulla. This potent topical anti-inflammatory combination is not ototoxic. It slows the intense inflammation and exudation found in middle ear disease. Corticosteroids reduce the amount and viscosity of the secretions from the inflamed mucous membrane in the bulla. Decreasing doses of systemic corticosteroids may be used for a few weeks during the recovery phase.

When a bacterial infection is the cause of the otitis media, injectable enrofloxacin (Baytril injection, Bayer) is added to the DMSO-fluocinolone solution (1 mL enrofloxacin added to 8 mL DMSO-fluocinolone), and 0.5 ml to 1.0 mL is infused into the bulla with the dog in lateral recumbency and the affected ear up. This positioning allows the medication to have prolonged contact with the inflamed tissue while the dog recovers from the anesthetic. After the dog awakens and turns its head to normal position, the medication in the tympanic bulla leaks into the horizontal canal.

Systemic antibiotics are chosen according to results of either culture and sensitivity testing of samples taken from the bulla or gram staining of the cytological samples from the bulla. Most of the *Pseudomonas, Staphylococcus,* and *Proteus* species commonly cultured from the ear are sensitive to the fluoroquinolones, which are therefore good first antibiotic choices. The higher enrofloxacin dosage regimens, 10 mg/kg bid or 20 mg/kg once daily, are preferred because of the higher initial antibiotic level that they achieve.

A common dilemma arises because systemic medications may not achieve tissue levels in the mucoperiosteum or tympanic cavity sufficient to kill organisms in the exudates, whereas topical medication may not gain access to the bulla. In otitis media, hyperemic, inflamed tissues may aid in transporting antimicrobial drugs from the blood into an otherwise inaccessible area. Some of the newer antibiotics that concentrate in inflammatory cells may be delivered directly to the site of inflammation.

Infusion of antibiotics directly into the clean tympanic bulla may achieve 50 to 100 times the antibiotic concentration provided by parenteral administration, but such an infusion cannot maintain prolonged therapeutic levels in the bulla and so must be repeated frequently. Instillation of antibiotic into the bulla is obviously impractical in an outpatient. Instillation of ear drops into the external ear canal may not even reach the bulla filled with mucus and pus. Many topical drugs are inactivated by the exudates or are not effective at the low pH found in the exudate. Pretreatment with trisEDTA at pH 8.0 helps improve the efficacy of topical antibiotics.

The use of fluoroquinolones may prove to solve this dilemma. When used at elevated doses, parenteral or oral fluoroquinolones can achieve tissue levels within the middle ear well above the minimum inhibitory concentrations (MICs) for most bacteria, including *Pseudomonas*. Topical fluoroquinolones infused directly into the bullae of hospitalized patients provide immediate therapeutic levels well in excess of the MIC, which may be more important than prolonged antibiotic levels. A new topical otic fluoroquinolone, ofloxacin, when used twice daily in children with bacterial otitis externa and suppurative otitis media, resulted in an 82% cure rate in 2 weeks.

Middle ear disease resulting from yeasts or fungi is rare but may require systemic antifungal drugs. Ketoconazole, itraconazole, or fluconazole can be used to treat middle ear disease. Itraconazole and fluconazole, although more expensive, may be better than ketoconazole at reaching the middle ear with oral administration.

After Resolution of Otitis Media

A large number of patients may actually continue to have otitis media even after the external ear canal disease wanes and the eardrum has healed (Fig. 8–16). One study of 23 dogs treated for otitis media in the clinic demonstrated that this phenomenon occurred in 82.6% of ears. The organisms isolated from samples obtained from the middle ear by myringotomy correlated with the bacteria isolated from samples from the horizontal ear canal in only 10% of the samples tested; in the other 90%, the isolated organisms were different. The epidermal tissue of the ear canal and the respiratory epithelium lining the bulla support different bacteria. Therefore, culture samples obtained by myringotomy are indicated in many cases of otitis media to determine the best antibiotic for treatment of otitis media.

Myringotomy

To diagnose these patients it is sometimes necessary to perform a myringotomy to get a culture and antibiotic sensitivity on the material trapped behind the eardrum. For the myringotomy, the patient is anesthetized and the external ear canal is thoroughly cleaned with a disinfectant such as dilute povidone-iodine. The ear canal is then dried using

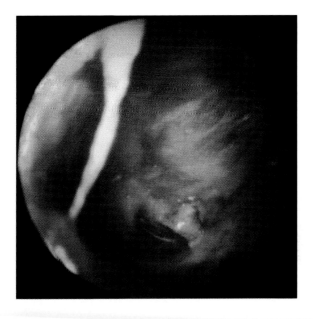

Figure 8-16

Healed eardrum in a 9-year-old Shetland sheepdog. After resolution of the bacterial infection and frequent middle ear suction procedures, the eardrum finally healed. Otitis media may still be present behind the healed eardrum.

suction. A sterile rigid polypropylene catheter is cut to a 60-degree angle with a surgery blade to provide a sharp point. A long spinal needle can also be used to puncture the eardrum. The tip of the cut catheter is advanced under good visualization and the pars tensa is punctured at either the 5 o'clock or 7 o'clock position in order to remain clear of the germinal epithelium overlying the manubrium of the malleus.

The catheter is advanced through the incised tympanic membrane, directed ventrally into the bulla, and gentle suction is used to retrieve any material within the bulla. If a spinal needle is used, the stylet is withdrawn prior to suctioning. If the bulla is dry, 1 or 2 ml of normal saline can be infused into the bulla and then immediately retrieved. This material is submitted for culture and antibiotic sensitivity. Cytology of this specimen may reveal Malassezia.

In the case of suppurative otitis media, myringotomy serves to decrease the fluid pressure behind the eardrum. The fluid escapes into the external ear canal, which must be periodically flushed to remove this debris.

Many eardrums heal only partially and a ring of granulation tissue develops. In most such cases, the bulla remains dry and the exudation from the mucoperiosteum subsides. Potentially ototoxic topical medications should be avoided in these cases. Frequent otoscopic examinations are essential in assessing patients with these features. If material continues to accumulate in the bulla, suctioning may need to be repeated at weekly or biweekly intervals to help remove exudates.

Surgical Treatment

In spite of concentrated efforts to treat otitis media medically, irreversible pathological changes often prevent cures. The chronically reactive tissues become resistant to medical treatment. Drugs cannot penetrate the tissues, but bacteria flourish in the crypts of epithelium and the sclerotic bone. Objectives of surgery in chronic unresponsive otitis media are (1) removing infected tissues from the bulla or external ear canal, (2) allowing drainage of exudates from the ventral part of the bulla, and (3) enabling local treatment of infection in the bulla.

Many cases of chronic, suppurative otitis media require lateral ear canal resection to allow the exudates produced within the inflamed bulla to drain out into the external ear canal and to provide adequate access to the middle ear for flushing.

Ventral bulla osteotomy for middle ear drainage is indicated when the external ear canal is normal but the middle ear remains actively inflamed or infected. This exposure also provides an opening for the surgeon to curette the infected mucoperiosteum. It is the preferred surgical approach for removal of nasopharyngeal polyps. A drain placed in the bulla that exits adjacent to the surgical incision in the neck provides an exit for flushing solutions that are infused into the bulla via the external canal.

Ablation of the vertical ear canal is indicated when the severe stenosis of the ear canal causes pressure to build up in the ear canal and bulla distal to the stenosis. Tumors, sclerosis, and hyperplastic tissue are removed along with the vertical ear canal cartilage in a funnel-shaped en bloc dissection. The cartilaginous portion of the horizontal canal may be also removed in this procedure. The objective is to remove enough tissue to restore patency to the lumen of the ear canal.

Total ear canal ablation and lateral bulla osteotomy are indicated when the cartilage of the ear canal has ossified and the resulting stenosis prevents the introduction of either medications or surgical instruments into the inflamed middle ear.

Surgical procedures used to drain exudates from the bulla may often be followed by complications such as wound dehiscence, sinus tract formation, abscess formation, and temporary facial nerve damage.

Conclusion

Owners of dogs with otitis media must be counseled by the veterinarian. They must understand that the chronic inflammatory changes in the middle ear do not subside immediately and treatment of these difficult cases can be very prolonged and may eventually require surgery.

Suggested Readings

Albino AP, Kimmelman CP, Parisier SC: Cholesteatoma: A molecular and cellular puzzle. Am J Otol 19:7–19, 1998.

Cole LK: Microbial flora and antimicrobial sensitivity patterns of isolated pathogens from the horizontal ear canal and middle ear in dogs with otitis media. J Am Vet Med Assoc 212:534–538, 1998.

Davidson EB, Brodie HA, Breznock EM: Removal of a cholesteatoma in a dog, using a caudal auricular approach. J Am Vet Med Assoc 211:1549–1553, 1997.

Lim DJ: Structure and function of the tympanic membrane: A review. Acta Otorhinolaryngol Belg 49:101–115, 1995.

Little CJL, Lane JG, Pearson GR, Gibbs C: Inflammatory middle ear disease of the dog: The clinical and pathological features of cholesteatoma, a complication of otitis media. Vet Rec 128:319–322, 1991.

Mansfield PD, Steiss JE, Boosinger TR, Marshall AE: The effects of four commercial ceruminolytic agents on the middle ear. J Am Anim Hosp Assoc 33:479–486, 1997.

Neer TM: Otitis media. Veterinary Learning Systems. Compend Cont Ed Pract Vet 4:410–418, 1982.

Vennix P, Kuijpers W: Keratinocyte differentiation in acquired cholesteatoma and perforated tympanic membranes. Arch Otolaryngol Head Neck Surg 122:825–832, 1996.

9

Ototoxicity of Topical Preparations

Philip D. Mansfield, DVM
Starr C. Miller, DVM

O *totoxicity* may be defined as substance-induced damage to or destructive effect on the structure and function of the ear. Ototoxicity after parenteral administration of certain substances is well documented. Parenterally induced ototoxicity results in injury to the endorgans of the vestibulocochlear nerve located in the inner ear that may result in minimal damage or may cause complete loss of auditory and vestibular function. The effects may be temporary or permanent. Agents that can result in ototoxicity when administered systemically are listed in Table 9–1.

Less well known is the potential for ototoxicity resulting from the use of topical agents. Although topical agents are generally accepted as safe to use in the presence of an intact tympanic membrane, damage may occur if medication enters the middle ear through a tympanic membrane perforation. When the tympanic membrane is perforated (secondary to infection and inflammation, as a result of a myringotomy, or iatrogenically), preparations applied topically to the external ear canal can enter the middle ear cavity and can be absorbed by the mucosa and the submucosa. Subsequently, there may be a local inflammatory response resulting in morphological and functional alteration of structures within the middle ear or the substance may penetrate the cochlear window (round window) and enter the inner ear. The primary sites of injury within the inner ear appear to be the sensorineural cells of the cochlea and the vestibular apparatus. Cochlear injury in animals is likely to go unnoticed until there is severe bilateral hearing loss. Vestibular injury may be inapparent or may result in signs such as head tilt, circling, nystagmus, and ataxia. The clinical signs manifested by the affected animal depend on the structures injured and the amount of injury sustained.

Alterations of the middle ear include serous or mucoid effusion, mucosal hyperplasia, formation of granulation tissue, erosion of the auditory ossicles, resorption of the osseous bulla, and deposition of new bone within the otic capsule. These morphological changes may lead to a conductive hearing loss that is incomplete and undetected.

Regardless of experimental evidence, because of discrepancy between the data and clinical experience, there remains controversy regarding the significance of topical ototoxicity and the relative safety of using topical otic preparations in dogs and cats. This discrepancy may reflect a lesser vulnerability for dogs and cats than observed for other species of laboratory animals used in ototoxicity studies. It is more likely that the adverse effects in pet animals are clinically inapparent and, therefore, are considered nonexistent. In other instances, clinical signs of toxicity may be regarded as sequelae of the primary disease.

Many factors may affect the development of ototoxicity and subsequent clinical signs. For example, the amount of a substance that actually

TABLE 9–1. Ototoxic Systemic Agents

Aminoglycoside antibiotics	Amikacin
	Dactinomycin
	Dibekacin
	Dihydrostreptomycin
	Framycetin
	Gentamicin
	Kanamycin
	Netilmicin
	Ribostamycin
	Sisomicin
	Streptomycin
	Tobramycin
Nonaminoglycoside antibiotics	Erythromycin
	Ristocetin
Diuretics	Acetazolamide
	Bumetanide
	Ethacrynic acid
	Furosemide
	Mannitol
Antineoplastic agents	Actinomycin C & D
	Bleomycin
	Carboplatin
	Cisplatin
	Mechlorethamine
	Vinblastine
	Vincristine
Miscellaneous agents	Arsenic compounds
	Chloroquine
	Danazol
	Gold salts
	Pentobarbital
	Potassium bromide
	Quinidine
	Quinine
	Salicylates

enters the middle ear and the absorption of that substance into the inner ear depends on the following factors:

- Length and shape of the external ear canal
- Size of the defect in the tympanic membrane
- Volume and viscosity of the applied substance
- Patency of the eustachian tube
- Presence of physical barriers obstructing passage to the round window
- Permeability of the round window membrane

In the healthy middle ear of experimental animals, the mucosa, including the layer of epithelial cells covering the round window, is very thin compared with the mucosa in ears affected by disease. The thickening of the mucosa, granulation tissue in the round window, and the presence of middle ear effusions may impede the penetration of substances to the inner ear. Conversely, it has been reported that with acute otitis media, the round window membrane becomes more permeable. Obviously, there remains uncertainty regarding the effects of middle ear inflammation on the potential for a substance to penetrate the inner ear.

Once a substance penetrates the round window, other factors govern its distribution in the fluid compartments of the inner ear and its accessibility to the sensory receptors. The concentration of the toxic substance and the duration of exposure have been shown to correlate with the severity of injury. The cumulative effects of repeated exposures may produce pathological changes that were initially inapparent. Age, anesthesia, preexisting cochlear or vestibular damage, and the additive effects of other ototoxic substances are factors that may potentiate ototoxicity. Familial susceptibility to ototoxicity occurs in humans.

Fifteen percent to 20% of all dogs suffer from otitis externa; 50% of dogs with chronic otitis externa have rupture of the tympanic membrane and concurrent otitis media. Because of the frequency of otitis externa, ototoxicity is more likely to occur in dogs as a result of topical application. Topical otic preparations that are routinely used in treating otitis externa contain a variety of potentially ototoxic antibiotics, antiseptics, fungicidal agents, ceruminolytic and cleaning agents, and solvents (Table 9–2). The potential for many of these preparations and their constituents to cause damage to the middle and inner ear has been documented in a variety of animal species.

Labels that warn against use of otic preparations in an animal with perforation of the tympanic membrane are at times dismissed. This situation may be attributable to lack of patient cooperation to allow examination of the ear without anesthesia, lack of client time or money to permit evaluation of the ear with the patient under anesthesia for a perceived minor problem, lack of visualization of the tympanic membrane without thorough cleaning of the ear canal, or other factors. Even when the tympanic membrane can be visualized with an otoscope, assessment

TABLE 9–2. Potentially Ototoxic Topical Agents

Aminoglycoside antibiotics: All	
Nonaminoglycoside antibiotics	Bacitracin*
	Chloramphenicol*
	Chlortetracycline*
	Colistin*
	Erythromycin
	Gramicidin*
	Hygromycin B
	Iodochlorhydroxyquinolone
	Minocycline
	Oxytetracycline*
	Pharmacetin
	Polymyxin B
	Tetracycline*
	Ticarcillin*
	Vancomycin
	Viomycin
Antiseptics	Acetic acid
	Benzalkonium chloride*
	Benzethonium chloride
	Cetrimide
	Chlorhexidine*
	m-Cresyl acetate
	Ethanol
	Iodine and iodophors
	Merthiolate
Antifungal agents	Amphotericin B*
	Griseofulvin*
Ceruminoluytic agents and solvents	Carbamide peroxide*
	Dimethyl formamide
	Dioctyl sodium sulfosuccinate*
	Ethanol
	Propylene glycol*
	Polyethylene glycol 400
	Triethanolamine
	Toluene
Miscellaneous agents	Cyclophosphamide
	Dapsone
	Detergents
	Dimethylsulfoxide
	Diphenylhydrazine
	Mercury
	Potassium bromide
	Triethyl tin bromide
	Trimethyl tin chloride

*Has an inflammatory effect on the middle ear.

is difficult. One cannot be certain that the tympanic membrane is intact unless pneumatic otoscopy or tympanometry is performed. Furthermore, some ototoxic preparations do not have a warning label. Nevertheless, there is risk of injury to the middle ear, inner ear, or both when any of the agents discussed in the next section are used in the external ear canal of an animal with a perforated tympanic membrane.

Ototoxic Substances

Antibiotics

Aminoglycoside Antibiotics

All of the aminoglycoside antibiotics have ototoxic properties. Toxicity has been attributed to aminoglycoside concentrations; these substances form in the perilymph and endolymph, subsequently destroying auditory and vestibular hair cells in a manner much like their effect on bacterial cells. It has also been reported that the aminoglycosides adversely affect the stria vascularis, resulting in secondary hair cell loss. Perhaps there is both primary and secondary damage to the hair cell; the actual mechanism remains uncertain.

At high dosages, all aminoglycoside antibiotics may affect both cochlear and vestibular function; however, specific compounds show a predilection for the cochlea (neomycin, kanamycin, and amikacin) or the vestibular apparatus (streptomycin and gentamicin). Studies in guinea pigs, chinchillas, cats, and humans have demonstrated a marked degree of topical aminoglycoside–induced ototoxicity. The hearing loss following aminoglycoside exposure may take up to 6 months to develop and may progress for up to 12 months after administration of the agent. Aminoglycoside-induced vestibular toxicity in humans is often described as a failure to fix on the horizon, with the sensation that distant stationary objects appear to move. These observations of ototoxicity in humans help to explain why it is difficult to assess cochlear and vestibular damage in animals.

Nonaminoglycoside Antibiotics

Other antibiotics that are ototoxic when applied to the middle ear cavity are listed in Table 9–2. Most of these drugs cause inflammation in the middle ear and osseous changes in the bulla.

Antiseptics

Antiseptic solutions infused into the middle ear through a perforated tympanic membrane can produce partial or total loss of vestibular function, cochlear function, or both. Commonly used ototoxic antiseptics are acetic acid, benzalkonium chloride, benzethonium chloride, chlorhexidine, ethanol, iodine, and iodophors.

Chlorhexidine has been incriminated as a highly ototoxic substance. In addition to damaging cochlear and vestibular hair cells, this agent may cause fibrosis and ossification in the middle ear and inner ear. Experimentally, chlorhexidine is ototoxic in rats, guinea pigs, and cats. Clinically, humans and dogs have exhibited immediate cochlear and vestibular dysfunction after instillation of chlorhexidine into the middle ear. At a referral institution, three cases of deafness in dogs subsequent to topical application of chlorhexidine prompted an investigation of that compound's ototoxicity in dogs (Merchant, 1993). In that study, no adverse effect was observed. Nevertheless, the investigator cautions against concluding that ototoxicity cannot result from the use of this compound. The United States Food and Drug Administration (FDA) has eliminated chorhexidine from use in otic preparations because of demonstrated ototoxicity.

Fungicidal Agents

Because pathogenic fungi, especially *Malassezia pachydermatis,* may be primary or secondary pathogens in otitis externa, fungicides and antiseptics that have fungicidal activity are frequently used topically in the ear. Some of these substances are potentially ototoxic. Amphotericin B placed in the middle ear provokes a mucosal inflammatory response. Griseofulvin produces severe cochlear hair cell loss as well as local mucosal inflammation when instilled into the middle ear.

All of the antiseptics that are used in the ear for their antimycotic activity (acetic acid, aqueous merthiolate, chlorhexidine, iodine, iodophors, and *m*-cresyl acetate) have been shown to have adverse effects on the middle or inner ear.

Ceruminolytic or Cleaning Agents

Examination of the external meatus and the tympanic membrane of the inflamed ear cannot be completed and effective treatment cannot be accomplished if the canal is occluded with cerumen or exudate. Cleaning is often performed with commercial preparations formulated to soften and emulsify the wax and lipids in the ear canal. The labels of only a few of these preparations bear warnings that the products should not be used if the animal's tympanic membrane is perforated. Safety studies have not been performed on all the otic cleaning preparations currently marketed, although some contain ingredients that are known to be ototoxic.

In a study of four commercial ceruminolytic preparations, performed by one of the authors (Mansfield et al, 1997), inflammation and hearing loss were induced by three of the preparations. Thirty-four of 42 animals suffered severe injury to the middle ear, inner ear, or both when any one of three compounds was placed in the middle ears of guinea pigs (N = 24) and dogs (N = 18). If these had been pet animals receiving routine care, it is unlikely that any clinical signs would have been observed, except in one dog that demonstrated a persistent head tilt, nystagmus, and marked postural reaction deficits. Upon close examination, a slight head tilt was observed for a brief time in 13 guinea pigs and one dog. Six of the guinea pigs with head tilt also exhibited nystagmus that resolved within 3 to 4 days of onset. Cochlear dysfunction (N = 31) was detected only by brain evoked auditory response (BAER); inflammatory changes remained inapparent until necropsy.

Miscellaneous Agents

Parasiticides, astringents, and carrier vehicles are constituents of many otic preparations. Parasiticidal otic preparations have been incriminated as a cause of eruptions in the external ear canal. It has been thought that ototoxicity occurs in small animals when antiparasitic drugs penetrate the middle ear via a ruptured tympanic membrane. However, controlled studies of the effects of parasiticides in the middle ear and inner ear have not been reported.

Astringents (lactic acid, malic acid, benzoic acid, salicylic acid, aluminum silicate, and aluminum acetate) are constituents of otic drying preparations. The safety of these compounds is unknown.

Propylene glycol, a carrier vehicle that is common to many otic preparations, causes granulation and ossification of the auditory bulla as well as morphological and functional changes in the cochlea. Polyethylene glycol 400 and dimethyl foramimide are other solvents that have been shown to have adverse effects on the middle ear mucosa and the organ of Corti. No reports on the effects of glycerin have been published. Glycerin does have physical and chemical properties similar to those of propylene glycol.

Safe Ototopical Agents

Ideally, any preparation that is used topically in the ear would be free of risk for adverse effects. Unfortunately, this is not always true, but a few agents have been reported to be nontoxic when applied to the external canal of an ear with a perforated tympanic membrane. These agents are listed in Table 9–3, but the authors provide no assurance of their safety, nor has the FDA approved all of these agents for topical use in the ear. Risk of adverse effects on the middle ear and inner ear must be assumed when any substance is applied to the external ear canal in the presence of a tympanic membrane perforation.

TABLE 9–3. Safe Ototopical Agents*

Antibiotics	Carbenicillin
	Ceftazidime
	Cefmenoxime
	Ciprofloxacin
	Enrofloxacin
	Fosfomycin
	Ofloxacin
	Penicillin G
Anti-inflammatory agents	Dexamethasone
	Triamcinolone
Antifungal agents	Clotrimazole
	Nystatin
	Tolnaftate
Ceruminolytic agents and solvents	Isopropyl myristate
	Squalane

*Generally regarded as safe on the basis of published reports.

Comments

Topical treatment has an important role in the management of otic disease. Some otic preparations are safe only in the external ear canal. When they are used in animals with tympanic membrane perforation, the normally protected middle ear may be exposed to agents that can cause an inflammatory response in the tympanic bulla or sensory dysfunction in the inner ear.

Only a small percentage of animals with tympanic membrane defects actually demonstrate clinical signs of ototoxicity. It is conceivable, however, that we do not fully appreciate the extent of injury that is sustained in many instances. Although the occurrence of topically induced ototoxicity is controversial, the risk of using potentially ototoxic agents in animals that may have perforation of the tympanic membrane should be acknowledged as a valid concern.

Preparations containing potentially ototoxic agents should be used judiciously in patients with tympanic membrane perforation only after the benefits and risks have been carefully considered. Using as little of a topical agent for as short a course as possible may reduce the risk. Few topical agents appear to be free of toxic effects, but ototoxic injury can be minimized or prevented by thoughtful selection of therapeutic agents, attention to risk factors, and careful patient monitoring if long-term use is necessary. Renewable prescriptions should not be given cavalierly.

References and Suggested Readings

Kuhweide R: Experimental evidence of ototoxicity of ear drops: A review of the literature. *Acta Otorhinolaryngol Belg* 49:293–298, 1994.

Mansfield PD: Ototoxicity in dogs and cats. *Compend Cont Ed Pract Vet* 12:331–337, 1990.

Mansfield PD, Steiss JE, Boosinger TR, et al: The effects of four commercial ceruminolytic agents on the middle ear. *J Am Anim Hosp Assoc* 33:479–486, 1997.

Merchant SR: Ototoxicity. *Vet Clin North Am Small Anim Pract* 24:971–980, 1994.

Merchant SR: Ototoxicity assessment of a chlorhexidine otic preparation in dogs. Prog Vet Neurol 4:72–75, 1993.

Pickrell JA, Oehme FW, Cash WC: Ototoxicity in dogs and cats. *Semin Vet* Med Surg (Small Anim) 8:42–49, 1993.

Rohn GN, Meyerhoff WL, Wright CG: Ototoxicity of topical agents. *Otolaryngol Clin North Am* 26:747–758, 1993.

10

Failure of Epithelial Migration: Ceruminoliths

Louis N. Gotthelf, DVM

The ear canal requires a clearance mechanism to remove the accumulation of dead cells, foreign debris, and wax. Without a physiological method of debris removal, large accumulations of material remain.

A number of different substances that may be found in the ear canal must be removed or they will result in significant accumulations within the canal. The ear canal is lined by stratified squamous epithelium in a constant state of growth, so desquamated surface epithelial cells must be removed. Sebaceous and apocrine glands produce ceruminous secretions, and in certain conditions, cerumen accumulation may be quite voluminous. The wax must be removed. Debris from within the ear canal, such as exudates from otitis externa, must be removed. Substances that gain access to the ear canal from outside the ear, such as plant material and accumulation of ear medications, must also be removed. How does the normal ear canal remove all of this accumulated debris?

Epithelial Migration

Fortunately, the ordered growth of the ear canal epithelium facilitates a clearing mechanism termed *epithelial migration*. Simply stated, the epithelium in the ear canal grows outward from the tympanic membrane toward the opening of the external ear canal. As the surface epithelial cells move, they carry along any debris on top of them. This physiological epithelial movement process may be demonstrated by placing India ink on the eardrum and observing its dispersal along the ear canal over several weeks. The rate of epithelial movement is slow, and in older animals and people, the rate becomes even slower. When the rate slows to the point of allowing accumulation of debris, the term *failure of epithelial migration* applies (Fig. 10–1). When this condition causes accumulation of substances within the ear canal, ear flushes and ceruminolytic agents play an important role in its management.

A simple squamous germinal epithelium lines the lateral surface of the tympanic membrane in the external ear canal, especially in the area of the handle of the malleus, the pars tensa. It has been hypothesized that these germinal cells differentiate into epithelial cells called *basal keratinocytes* with very loose attachments to the basement membrane.

Basal keratinocytes migrate radially on the surface of the eardrum, becoming continuous with the epithelium of the external ear canal. Evidence of this phenomenon has been gained from studying the resultant migration of squamous epithelium into the middle ear cavity following myringotomy performed at the periphery of the eardrum.

Migration of epithelium from the pars tensa of the tympanic membrane toward the annular region of the eardrum to the epithelium of the horizontal canal provides a clearance mechanism for the migratory ke-

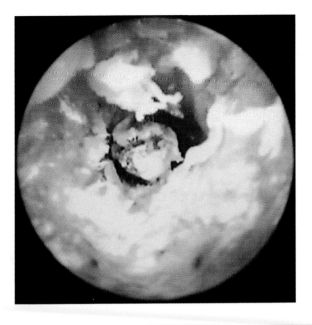

Figure 10–1

Failure of epithelial migration. During examination of the ear in a 14-year-old mixed-breed dog, flakes of dry epithelium and wax were seen lying along the ear canal wall. The ear clearance mechanism has failed in this patient, allowing epithelial cells to accumulate.

ratinocytes that result from normal stratified squamous epithelial physiology in the external ear canal. Cerumen, which covers the keratinocytes, is cleared from the ear canal along with the migrating epithelium.

Besides playing a role in protecting the ear canal as a mechanical barrier to environmental substances, the keratinocytes have been shown to possess immune functions. Interleukin-1 (IL-1) is stored in keratinocytes. When these cells are damaged, IL-1 is released, stimulating other cells to release more IL-1, and a cascade of immunological events results in the migration of granulocytes, monocytes, and macrophages into the site of damage. When an area of the ear canal has been denuded by trauma or ulcer formation, loss of this protective immune mechanism allows unchecked bacterial colonization, favoring development of otitis externa.

Failure of Epithelial Migration

Damage to the germinal epithelium of the eardrum from infection or ear mite infestation results in damage to the keratinocytes on the surface of the tympanic membrane (Fig. 10–2). During the healing process, fibrosis

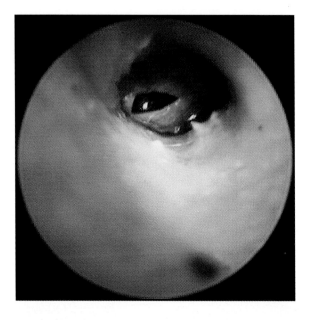

Figure 10–2

The patient, a 3-year-old cat, was presented with severe ear mite infestation. The ear canal was gently flushed with warmed dilute povidone-iodine solution to remove the ear mite debris. After cleaning, the eardrum can be seen to have a hole in it. It is hypothesized that damage to the eardrum's epithelial surface prevents radial movement of superficial keratinocytes, often resulting in waxy accumulation on the eardrum.

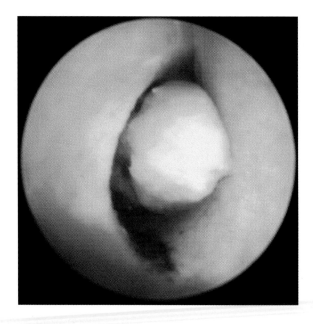

Figure 10–3

Soft wax ball at the eardrum. The eardrum is visible at the ventral portion of the wax ball, between it and the horizontal ear canal.

158

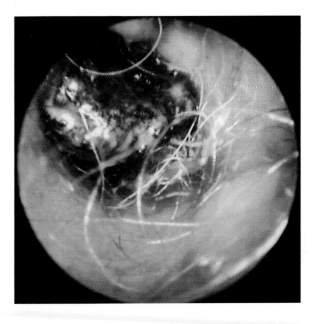

Figure 10–4

A hard concretion at the eardrum of a 15-year-old poodle. Note the hairs included in the ceruminolith matrix and the normal appearance to the horizontal canal epithelium.

may cause permanent changes to the tympanic membrane. Normal epithelial migration may be disrupted. Failure of epithelial migration may result in the accumulation of flakes of skin in the ear canal. More often, however, wax and keratin accumulate at the base of the eardrum and form either soft wax plugs (Fig. 10–3) or large, hard concretions called *ceruminoliths* (Fig. 10–4). To find them when examining the ear canals with an otoscope, the veterinarian should follow the bend in the ear cartilage and look in the horizontal canal toward the eardrum. Ceruminoliths are found lying along the floor of the horizontal ear canal.

Ceruminoliths

If the dog in which a ceruminolith is developing has a large number of hairs originating from around the annulus of the tympanic membrane, the hairs are included in the matrix of the ceruminolith. As the concretion moves, in response to head movement and gravity, these hairs are pulled and may cause significant discomfort. Bristly, thick hairs, as found in some dogs, that become involved in ceruminolith formation may irritate the ear canal lining and may also cause discomfort (Fig. 10–5). In the

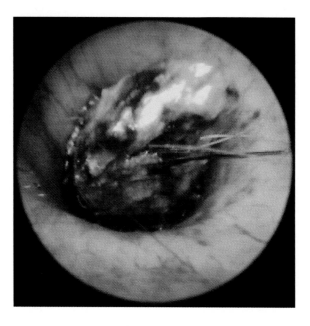

Figure 10–5

This large ceruminolith in a German shepherd illustrates the inclusion of bristly hairs in the wax ball. In this photo, the thick hairs are touching the horizontal ear canal wall and causing discomfort. The horizontal ear canal's epithelium appears normal.

author's experience, these conditions are often found in dogs and cats with a history of previously resolved ear disease. When ceruminoliths occur, they are usually seen in an ear without evidence of other disease.

When epithelial migration is prevented from continuing, the keratinocytes on the eardrum form layers on top of each other and are pushed backward toward the eardrum. Over time, the net effect is significant accumulation of desquamation products that cannot clear away from the eardrum and out of the ear canal. Cerumen and hairs mix into the heap.

These accumulations can become quite large, some of them measuring 1 to 2 inches in length. Although innocuous in appearance, ceruminoliths plugging the horizontal ear canal diminish hearing. In certain head positions, the weight of the ceruminolith pushes against the eardrum and may cause increased air pressure within the middle ear cavity, leading to signs of vestibular disease (Fig. 10–6).

Otoscopic examination of a ceruminolith reveals that there is a base attached to the eardrum, with the body of the mass freely movable and unattached to the surrounding ear canal. The tips of long hairs may be seen on the surface. In many cases the peripheral portion of the pars tensa can be visualized.

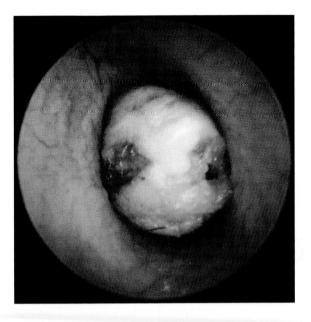

Figure 10–6

Soft wax ball. The owner of a 4-year-old cat presented the animal for diminished hearing and a head tilt. The history revealed that the cat had had severe recurrent ear mite infestations as a kitten.

Removal

The softer wax balls can be curetted or flushed out of the ear canal after treatment with a ceruminolytic agent such as dioctyl sodium sulfosuccinate. Warmed flush solutions help soften the waxy debris, and sometimes, careful suction with a large suction catheter aids in their removal (Fig. 10–7).

To remove a hardened concretion type of ceruminolith requires the use of a grasping forceps. The use of a video otoscope (Video Vetscope, MedRx, Inc., Seminole, FL) facilitates this process because the veterinarian can see the ceruminolith clearly on the video monitor. The endoscopic grasping tool, which is inserted through the biopsy channel of the video otoscope, can be carefully placed to grasp and remove the mass (Fig. 10–8).

After removal of these concretions, the tympanic membrane often looks abnormal. Small holes in the tympanum may be present because the epithelium is eroded along with the concretion as it is removed (Fig. 10–9). These small holes heal rapidly (Fig. 10–10).

If the eardrum was previously ruptured and a ceruminolith developed as a consequence, the healing tympanic epithelium may be in the middle of

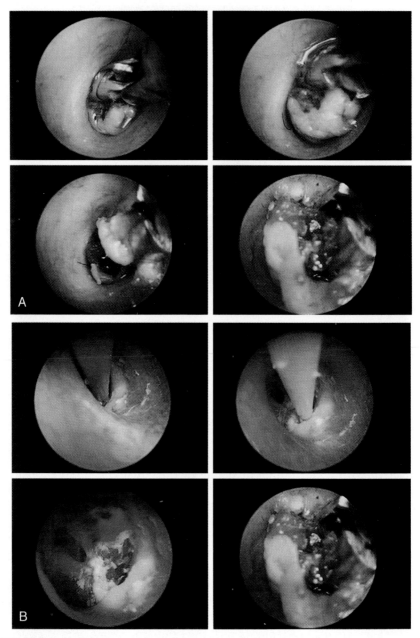

Figure 10–7

A, Removal of the soft wax ball from the cat in Figure 10–6. The mass was grasped with an endoscopic forceps. Because the wax was quite soft and malleable, the endoscopic graspers were ineffective at removing the wax. *B*, The ear was treated with a ceruminolytic and flushed with warmed dilute povidone-iodine solution. The soft wax was flushed from the ear, and small pieces of remaining debris were carefully suctioned off the surface of the eardrum.

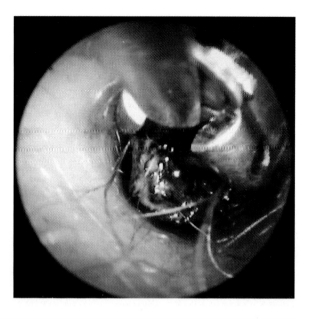

Figure 10–8

Endoscopic grasping forceps are used to remove the large, hard ceruminolith shown in Figure 10–4.

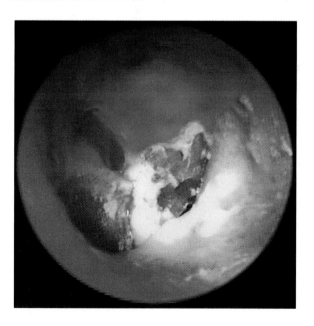

Figure 10–9

After removal of the wax plug from the cat in Figure 10–6, the eardrum was closely examined. A roughened surface and a small hole in the 5 o'clock position can be seen.

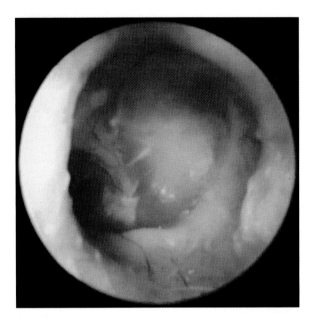

Figure 10–10

Close-up view of the eardrum from the cat in Figure 10–9 1 month after removal of the wax ball. The eardrum has healed and is almost normal in appearance. The cat was asymptomatic on this recheck visit.

a ceruminolith. When the concretion is removed, the eardrum is torn away, and a large direct communication to the tympanic bulla results. If detergent flush solutions were used for removal of the ceruminolith, copious saline flushes are used to remove these ototoxic substances (Figs. 10–11 and 10–12).

Older animals may have large accumulations of debris in the ear canals, because the epithelial migration process is quite slow in such animals. Occasional ear flushes may be required to augment the physiological cleaning process in these patients.

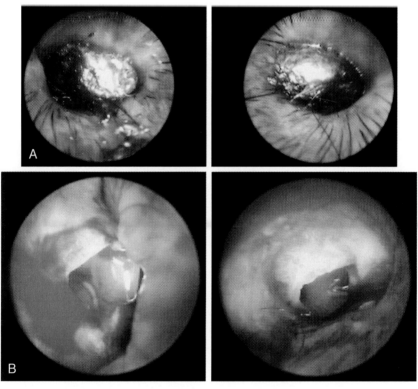

Figure 10–11

A, Bilateral ceruminoliths were identified in a 7-year-old mixed-breed dog with diminished hearing. *B,* The ceruminoliths were grasped with the endoscopic forceps and carefully removed. Both eardrums were ruptured, which may have resulted because each eardrum was involved in the matrix of the ceruminolith.

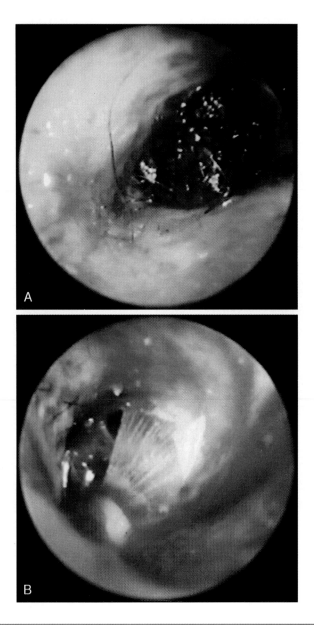

Figure 10–12

A, The patient, a 3-year-old German shepherd, was examined because of a painful ear. The affected ear was not being carried in the erect position. Examination of the ear canal revealed a wax plug at the level of the eardrum. *B,* The wax plug was grasped with the endoscopic forceps and carefully extracted. After the ear canal was flushed and dried, a partial tear of the eardrum could be seen. Mucus and pus consistent with otitis media are present under the cerumen plug.

Suggested Readings

Michaels I, Soucek S: Development of the stratified squamous epithelium of the human tympanic membrane and external ear canal: The origin of auditory epithelial migration. Am J Anat 184:334–344, 1989.

Smelt G, Stoney P, Weinberger J, Hawke M: Sequelae of experimental tympanic and inferior wall perforations: The double meaning of epithelial migration. J Otolaryngol 20:171–176, 1991.

11

Healing of the Ruptured Eardrum

Louis N. Gotthelf, DVM

Veterinarians are often faced with the problem of ruptured eardrums. It is difficult to assess the eardrum in a small animal because most otoscopes do not provide good lighting or adequate magnification. Many cases of otitis externa result in an ear canal that is inflamed, stenotic, and full of exudates that impede the visual determination of the integrity of the eardrum (Fig. 11–1).

Causes of Rupture

Tympanic membrane perforation occurs in dogs and cats for a variety of reasons, the most common being otitis externa. Otitis media results from the destructive effects of proteolytic enzymes on the thin epithelial layers of the membrane. These enzymes are released from bacteria, inflammatory cell degradation, and ulcerations along the ear canal produced as a result of otitis externa and then gain access to the sensitive respiratory lining of the tympanic bulla through the perforation.

Traumatic perforations of the tympanic membrane also occur as the result of either excessive fluid pressure achieved during flushing of the

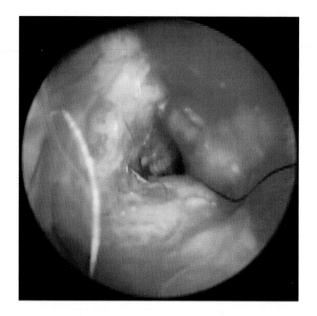

Figure 11–1

This eardrum of a 10-year-old German shepherd is ruptured. Copious mucoid debris filled the ear canal. The ear canal is edematous, and the eardrum cannot be visualized. Flush solution drained from the dog's nose and throat during the flushing process, confirming that the eardrum was not visible and the eustachian tube was open.

ear canal or traumatic use of instruments during cleaning of the ear canal (Fig. 11–2). Myringotomy, a traumatic perforation of the eardrum, may be iatrogenic or may be intentionally induced in therapy for otitis media.

Cats with respiratory disease may rupture their eardrums through sneezing. Increased air pressure builds within the eustachian tube during the violent act of sneezing, and that air pressure is transmitted through the eustachian tube to the middle ear cavity. When the pressure in the tympanic bulla exceeds 300 mm Hg, the eardrum ruptures (Fig. 11–3).

Rarely, ascending respiratory infections in dogs and cats resulting in suppurative otitis media may cause fluid pressure buildup inside the tympanic bulla. Without an exit point for the fluid, the increasing pressure within the tympanic cavity weakens the tympanic membrane, resulting in perforation. Children often suffer from this painful condition and require insertion of ventilation tubes in the eardrum to equalize the pressures between the tympanic bulla and the ear canal. In dogs and cats, myringotomy is indicated to relieve the pressure.

Nasopharyngeal polyps found in dogs and cats either grow along the eustachian tube toward the oropharynx or enlarge into the tympanic

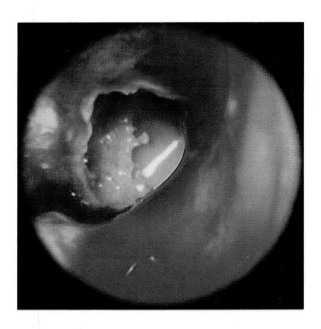

Figure 11–2

Traumatic myringotomy created by the use of a cotton-tipped applicator that was pushed too far into the horizontal canal.

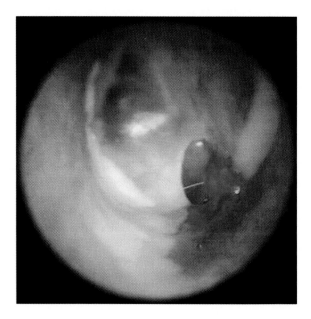

Figure 11–3

The patient, a young kitten with upper respiratory disease, was presented to the veterinarian with the complaints of sneezing and blood coming from the ear canal. Close examination of the eardrum reveals an acute perforation caused by increased air pressure within the bulla.

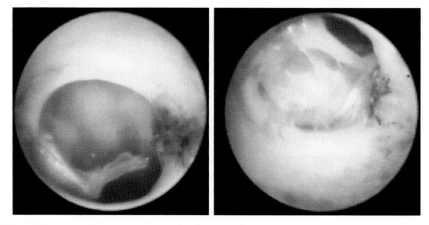

Figure 11–4

Left, Normal eardrum and tympanic bulla of a cat. *Right,* A polyp mass growing within the tympanic bulla pushing against the eardrum.

bulla. A large polyp within the tympanic bulla pushes against the eardrum, creating pressure necrosis, and its continued growth results in the ultimate destruction of the tympanic membrane (Fig. 11–4).

Healing Process

Unless the structures associated with the eardrum are completely destroyed, the eardrum attempts to heal. The mechanism for healing of a ruptured eardrum requires the presence of an adequate blood supply and a viable germinal epithelium. Regrowth of the eardrum depends on these vital structures, so the ability of the eardrum to heal is determined by the extent of the damage to them.

As discussed elsewhere, the germinal epithelium for the epidermal layer of the tympanic membrane is located in the area of the manubrium of the malleus and grows radially toward the annulus of the tympanic membrane from that location. Vascular supply to the germinal epithelium is derived from the blood vessels branching from the *pars flaccida* along the "vascular strip." If the malleus is preserved and the vascular strip is not compromised, the process of healing can continue (Fig. 11–5).

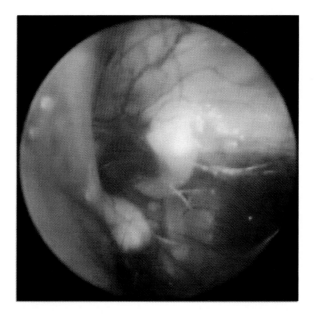

Figure 11–5

Prominent blood vessels in the pars flaccida. These blood vessels supply oxygen to the eardrum during the repair process.

The mechanism of healing in experimentally induced acute perforations of the eardrum has been studied in the dog. Tympanic membranes were perforated using a technique of subtotal myringectomy or by electrocautery. In these experiments, the attachment of the malleus to the tympanic membrane and vascular strip were preserved. Tympanic membrane healing was observed in all dogs otoscopically. The time required for complete regeneration of the ruptured eardrum ranged from 3 weeks to 4 months.

Cytological studies of how the tympanic membrane heals reveal that around the perforation border, keratinocytes on the external surface of the eardrum begin to proliferate. At the same time, fibrous connective tissue cells from the middle layer proliferate. The inner mucosal epithelial layer differentiates into ciliated and secretory cells only at the perforation border and cooperates with the proliferated keratinocytes to close the perforation. The superficial epithelial layers of the eardrum appear to be effective at rapidly moving toward the tympanic membrane perforation to form a temporary patch, but it is the slower-moving basal epithelial cells that are involved in permanent closure of the perforation (Fig. 11–6).

The intensity of this process may be directly proportional to the oxygenation provided to the cells by the intact vasculature. Vascular compromise or ischemia may impede tympanic membrane healing. Experimentally, in rats, aeration of the ruptured eardrum with increased oxygen concentrations resulted in acceleration of the healing process. This finding may have clinical implications in a patient in which the ear canal is stenotic and the eardrum is ruptured. Decreased ventilation of the ear canal may slow the healing rate.

The effects of naturally occurring otitis externa or otitis media on the tympanic membrane are different from those of experimentally produced perforations of the tympanic membrane. Progressive pathological changes interfere with the natural healing ability of the tympanic membrane. Inflammation, excessive fibrosis, tympanosclerosis, and hyperkeratosis are frequently found in and around the eardrum. Keratinized epithelial proliferation at the edge of the perforation often grows inward and localizes on the medial side of the tympanic membrane. A thick keratin layer protrudes into the middle ear at the periphery of a permanent perforation.

Otitis Media Prevents Healing

Otitis media is a highly secretory condition. Copious mucus results from the increased number and activity of goblet cells lining the tympanic bulla. Purulent exudates result from inflammation within the middle ear. The fluid may be thin and serous or thick and mucopurulent. The accumulation of mucus and pus creates a high fluid pressure between the

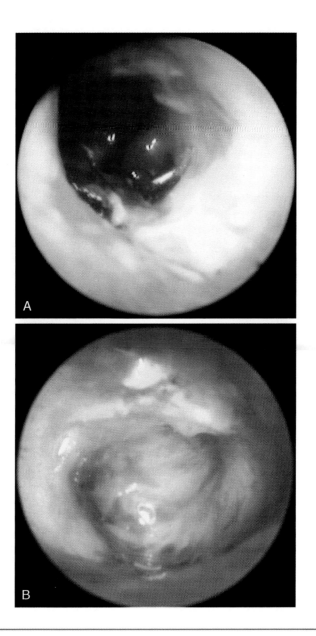

Figure 11–6

A, Chronic otitis media and ruptured eardrum in a 12-year-old Sheltie that was present for 6 months prior to treatment. *B,* Four months after treatment for the otitis media, the eardrum has healed.

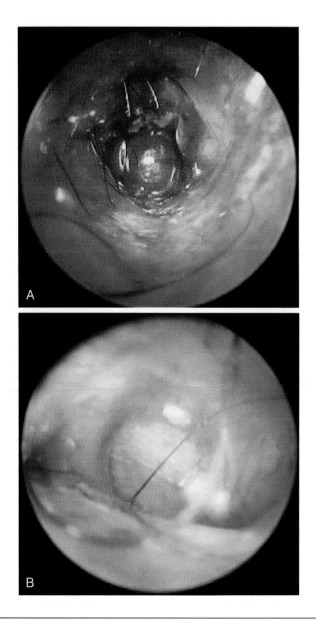

Figure 11–7

A, Severe mucopurulent discharge from the ear in *Pseudomonas* otitis externa/media in an 8-year-old Shih Tzu. The eardrum was not visible. *B,* After 6 months of treatment consisting of systemic and topical enrofloxacin, periodic middle ear flushes, trisEDTA ear flushes at home by the owners, and intermittent topical corticosteroids, the eardrum has healed.

middle ear cavity and the horizontal canal of the external ear canal. When the eustachian tube is inflamed or the exudate is very viscous, the fluid escapes from the middle ear cavity along the path of least resistance, which is through any perforation in the eardrum, and moves into the external ear canal. For healing of the tympanic membrane to progress, the mucus and pus must be removed from the bulla and ear canal (Fig. 11–7).

Effective treatment for otitis media diminishes production of mucopurulent fluid. Until there is a reduction in the amount of fluid produced by the mucoperiosteum, any attempt at eardrum healing is negated by the constant flow of fluid through the perforation. Treatment for otitis externa reduces the quantity and alters the chemical composition of the exudates that move distally along the ear canal toward the eardrum and decreases the amount of proteolytic enzymes acting to destroy the new epithelium that is attempting to heal the eardrum.

Depending on the severity of the otitis externa or otitis media, lysis of the malleus bone may be evident, and the germinal centers overlying this important structure destroyed. Extensive fibrosis may be present in the *pars flaccida* and around the annulus of the eardrum, occluding the vascular supply to the eardrum and leading to ischemia (Fig. 11–8). In either case, the essential components for eardrum healing are removed and a chronic perforation remains.

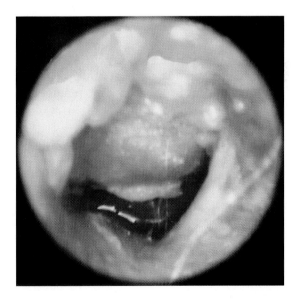

Figure 11–8

Chronic otitis media with extensive granulation tissue and fibrosis causing ischemia to the eardrum. The affected dog has permanent chronic otitis media.

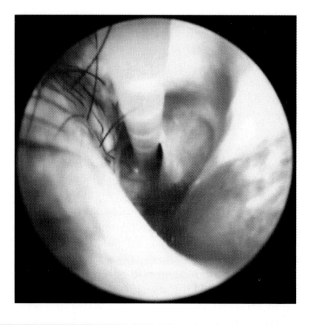

Figure 11–9

Chronic perforation of the tympanic membrane. A ring of hyperkeratosis surrounds the un-healed eardrum, allowing free access to the tympanic bulla. This dog had its ears flushed during grooming; 4 days later, the ear canal was full of mucus. The tip of the open-ended tomcat catheter is suctioning mucus from the middle ear.

Even if the otitis media is successfully treated and resolved, the eardrum may not heal completely closed. Often, a ring of hyperkeratotic epidermis surrounds the hole in the tympanic membrane; this condition represents a permanent perforation (Fig. 11–9). Any substance in the external ear canal, such as flush solution, exudates, loose hairs, epithelial cells, cerumen, or ototoxic otic drugs, can enter the middle ear and initiate an inflammatory response. Bacteria and yeasts gain access to the middle ear and provoke infection. Dogs with a permanent perforation of the tympanic membrane should not swim or get water in their ears. Veterinarians and groomers should be aware of this condition to ensure that no ototoxic ear cleaner or ototoxic topical medication enters the ears; otherwise, frequent flare-ups of otitis media result.

Chronic, persistent perforations of the tympanic membrane are common in people. The standard treatment is myringoplasty. This procedure is not performed in cats or dogs, however. An ongoing area of intense research is to identify substances that may be applied topically to the perforation to institute closure.

Suggested Readings

Boedts D: Tympanic membrane perforations. Acta Otorhinolaryngol Belg 49:149–158, 1995.

Caye-Tomasen P: Changes in goblet cell density in rat middle ear mucosa in acute otitis media. Am J Otol 16:75–82, 1995.

Clymer MA: The effects of keratinocyte growth factor on healing of tympanic membrane perforations. Laryngoscope 106:280–285, 1996.

Gotthelf LN: Secondary otitis media: An often overlooked condition. Canine Pract 20:14–20, 1995.

Koba K: Epidermal migration and healing of the tympanic membrane: An immunohistochemical study of cell proliferation using bromodeoxyuridine labelling. Ann Otol Rhinol Laryngol 104:218–225, 1995.

Little CJL, Lane JG, Pearson GR: Inflammatory middle ear disease of the dog: The pathology of otitis media. Vet Rec 128:293–296, 1991.

Mattson C: Myringosclerosis caused by increased oxygen concentration in traumatized tympanic membranes: Experimental study. Ann Otol Rhinol Laryngol 104:625–631, 1995.

Somers TH: Histology of the perforated tympanic membrane and its muco-epithelial junction. Clin Otolaryngol 22:162–166, 1997.

Steiss JE, Boosinger TR, Wright JC, Pillai SR: Healing of experimentally perforated tympanic membranes demonstrated by electrodiagnostic testing and histopathology. J Am Anim Hosp Asso 28:307–310, 1992.

Truy E: Chronic tympanic membrane perforation: An animal model. Am J Otol 16:222–225, 1995.

12

Ceruminous Otitis Externa

Norma White-Weithers, MS, DVM

Histopathology of the External Ear Canal

The epithelium of the external auditory meatus is composed of components similar to those of normal skin. The stratum corneum is the outermost layer, and keratinocytes make up this layer of squamous anuclear cells. There are no rete ridges in the epithelium of the ear canal. The sebaceous glands are the outermost glands and become progressively more numerous deeper into the meatus. Underlying the sebaceous glands are simple coiled tubular apocrine glands called *ceruminous glands* with ducts that open directly into hair follicles or onto the surface of the ear canal. During inflammatory reactions, sebaceous glands become hyperactive and hyperplastic, and the ceruminous glands become dilated, thickened, and filled with secretions. Under normal physiological conditions, ceruminous secretions *(cerumen)* combine with sebum produced by the sebaceous glands and epidermal debris to form *earwax*, the normal secretion of the ear.

Etiology of Ceruminous Otitis

When ceruminous glands and sebaceous glands of the ear canal become chronically irritated, the result is cystic dilation of ceruminous glands and hyperplasia and increased activity of the overlying sebaceous glands. The excessive amount of cerumen produced by ceruminous glands forms a favorable medium for the growth of secondary bacteria and yeast. These organisms, which are part of the normal flora of the ear, include *Pseudomonas* species, *Proteus* species, and *Malassezia pachydermatis*. With improper drainage and lack of air circulation (due to pendulous ears in some breeds), there may be excessive growth of these organisms within the ear canal. In most cases of ceruminous otitis, the epidermal hyperplasia and inflammatory reaction occlude the external ear canal, making visual examination difficult. In both the dog and cat, hyperplasia of the ear canal can simulate neoplastic conditions, leading to misdiagnoses and improper treatment. When hyperplasia does not respond to treatment and hardening of the ear canal ensues, surgical intervention is often the treatment of choice. Surgical opening of the ear canal allows proper drainage. The identification and treatment of underlying infections are important for surgical success.

Ceruminous otitis is inflammation of glandular structures of the ear canal with subsequent excessive epidermal proliferation and otitis externa that will require medical or surgical management. The causes of ceruminous otitis are many, and each condition is accompanied by other dermatological or systemic manifestations.

Disorders of Keratinization

Primary Idiopathic Seborrhea

Ceruminous otitis can be due to an inherited or acquired keratinization defect. Inherited disorders include idiopathic primary seborrhea, which is commonly seen in West Highland white terriers, American Cocker spaniels, English Springer spaniels, bassett hounds, Irish setters, Dachshunds, Chinese Shar Peis, and German shepherds. Primary idiopathic seborrhea, epidermal dysplasia of the West Highland white terrier, and lichenoid-psoriasiform dermatosis of English Springer spaniels are examples of primary keratinization defects with ceruminous otitis externa. Secondary or acquired keratinization defects include vitamin A–responsive dermatosis, zinc-responsive dermatosis, and fatty acid deficiency.

The epidermis of the canine ear canal undergoes proliferation, differentiation, and desquamation, with renewal of the viable epidermis in approximately 22 days. In American Cocker spaniels that have idiopathic primary seborrhea, the proliferative, differentiative, and desquamative stages take an average of 8 days. This rapid turnover of epidermal cells increases the renewal stage that will produce seborrhea (manifested as seborrheic dermatitis, ceruminous otitis, or both). This defect in differentiation may include hyperkeratosis or hypokeratosis and dyskeratosis.

Clinical Signs. The clinical signs of primary and secondary ceruminous otitis are the same and can be diagnosed only on the basis of response to therapy. In-depth clinical and diagnostic evaluations are mandatory for animals presented with chronic ceruminous otitis. These animals usually have other primary or secondary dermatological manifestations.

Clinical signs can be mild or chronic, with secondary bacterial or *Malassezia* infections complicating the primary problem. Ears with ceruminous otitis are malodorous and there is often secondary epidermal hyperplasia of the ear canal that may occlude the auditory meatus. Other presenting signs are usually generalized, focal to multifocal seborrheic dermatitis with secondary bacterial or *Malassezia* infections.

Animals with moist pendulous ears and poor ventilation, in the author's experience, are presented more often with chronic ceruminous otitis that requires generalized anesthesia for proper ear examination. Examination of such animals under generalized anesthesia allows the clinician to thoroughly visualize, clean, and obtain biopsy specimens from the ear.

A biopsy is often necessary to differentiate chronic epidermal hyperplasia with chronic ceruminous otitis from ceruminous gland tumors. Secondary bacterial and *Malassezia* infections respond when the underlying cause is properly treated. If there is no response, evaluation should consist of bacterial and fungal culture and sensitivity testing.

Diagnosis. Histological evaluation of noninfected seborrheic areas usually supports a diagnosis of primary seborrhea. After identification of secondary invaders and appropriate medical management, diagnosis is most frequently confirmed by response to treatment.

Treatment. Because ceruminous otitis is only the manifestation of a more serious problem, finding the underlying cause should be the clinician's primary goal. Treatment of primary seborrhea should attempt to control the disease rather than produce a complete cure. Treatment of the ears should focus on (1) control of secondary infections and production of scales and crust and (2) reduction of inflammation. Frequent ear cleaning with appropriate topical medication can control the odor associated with this condition. Steroids, cytotoxic drugs, and retinoic acid have variable effects. Results with the use of synthetic retinoid (etretinate) in the Cocker spaniel and other breeds to treat idiopathic seborrheas are disappointing. In the Cocker spaniel, there was a reduction of scales, crust, and alopecia, but the ceruminous otitis was not responsive to this therapy. Etretinate therapy was less effective in other breeds affected with this condition.

Endocrine Dermatosis

The most common endocrine diseases associated with ceruminous otitis are hypothyroidism and hyperadrenocorticism.

Hypothyroidism

Breeds with a predilection for hypothyroidism are golden retrievers, Alaskan malamutes, chow chows, Boxers, English bulldogs, Chinese Shar Peis, Great Danes, Afghan hounds, Doberman pinschers, Newfoundlands, dachshunds, and Cocker spaniels. Hypothyroidism in cats is extremely rare.

Etiology. The causes of hypothyroidism are classified as primary, secondary, tertiary, or congenital. Examples of causes of primary hypothyroidism are lymphocytic thyroiditis, thyroid atrophy, thyroid gland hyperplasia, neoplasia, and thyroid cell destruction due to radioactive iodine treatment or antithyroid drug therapy. Secondary hypothyroidism in the dog is the result of pituitary destruction and malformation or suppression of thyrotrophic cell function. There are no known causes of canine tertiary hypothyroidism. Defect in iodine organification and thyroid gland dysgenesis are the two most common causes of congenital hypothyroidism in the dog.

Clinical Signs. Thyroid hormone is an important regulator in the body's metabolic function. A deficiency causes a decrease in normal cellular metabolic functions of the body. The clinical signs of hypothyroidism in the dog are extremely variable, being those of metabolic, dermatologic, reproductive, neuromuscular, ocular, gastrointestinal, cardiovascular, and hematological disorders.

Serum and cutaneous fatty acid concentrations are affected by thyroid hormones. Thyroid hormones stimulate the synthesis, mobilization, and degradation of lipids, with the most dramatic effect being a decrease in degradation. This may present as an increase in serum low-density lipoprotein (LDL).

Thyroid hormone raises sebum production needed for the normal lipogenesis and synthesis of sterol by keratinocytes and increases cutaneous linoleic acid, with a decrease in gamma-linolenic and arachidonic acid concentrations. The decrease in arachidonic acid concentration alters epidermal proliferation. This alteration is responsible for the seborrhea, seborrheic dermatitis, and ceruminous otitis so often present in hypothyroid dogs. This may be the only presenting sign in a hypothyroid dog. The dryness or greasiness associated with the alteration of cutaneous fatty acid level can manifest as a dry or a greasy form of seborrhea.

Secondary bacterial and *Malassezia* infections are complicating factors in ceruminous otitis and can be a dermatological nightmare if not treated properly. Other dermatological abnormalities in dogs with hypothyroidism are myxedema, thin skin, hyperkeratosis, seborrheic ear pinnae, pyoderma, symmetrical or patchy endocrine alopecia, and various degrees of hyperpigmentation. Pruritus is often present with secondary bacterial or *Malassezia* infection.

Diagnosis and Treatment. The resolution of the ceruminous otitis largely depends on the proper diagnosis and control of hypothyroidism. History and physical examination findings are important in diagnosis of hypothyroidism. A complete blood count, serum biochemistry profile, urinalysis, and thyroid stimulation test are some of the few laboratory tests used to diagnose hypothyroidism.

Epidermal hyperplasia and pain often occur in the treatment of ceruminous otitis. Topical steroid preparations are useful in controlling pain and inflammation and reducing epidermal hyperplasia. Because steroids affect baseline thyroid levels, a thyroid stimulation test should precede the use of this therapy.

Hyperadrenocorticism

Bilateral adrenocortical hyperplasia due to pituitary adenomas is the most common cause of hyperadrenocorticism in the dog. The excessive production of steroid by the adrenal gland results in systemic as well as dermatological abnormalities. The prolonged exogenous use of oral, intra-muscular, or intravenous (and possibly otic and ophthalmic) cortico-steroids causes hyperadrenocorticism; other causes are adrenal adeno-mas and carcinomas.

The cutaneous manifestations of excessive serum cortisol are:

- Alopecia
- Failure or slowness of hair growth after clipping
- Thin skin
- Pyoderma
- Seborrhea
- Comedone formation
- Bruising
- Striae formation

Seborrheic dermatitis may manifest as ceruminous otitis with secondary bacterial or *Malassezia* infections.

Glucocorticoids inhibit epidermal proliferation and sebum production through antimitotic, protein-catabolic, and antienzymatic effects. The de-crease in hair growth is manifested clinically as bilateral symmetrical or moth-eaten–like alopecia. The antimetabolic and antiproliferative effects on fibroblasts are evident as poor wound healing. There is also an in-crease in susceptibility to infections. Because animals with hyperadreno-corticism show signs of secondary hypothyroidism, clinical signs of sebor-rhea and skin infection may be exaggerated by the dermatological effects of low thyroid levels.

The combination of seborrhea and bacterial or *Malassezia* infections can manifest as ceruminous otitis, which is not as common in the cat as in the dog.

Diagnosis and Treatment. Diagnosis of hyperadrenocorticism is based on history, results of complete blood count, serum biochemistry, uri-nalysis, adrenocorticotropic hormone (ACTH) stimulation test, and ultra-sonographic and radiographic findings. Because steroids affect thyroid levels, a thyroid stimulation test is part of the diagnostic plan. Treatment of otitis externa secondary to hyperadrenocorticism depends on proper di-agnosis and treatment of the hyperadrenocorticism. Any secondary bac-terial or *Malassezia* infection should also be treated.

Other Endocrine Dermatoses

Other causes of endocrine dermatosis are Sertoli cell tumors, seminoma, interstitial cell tumor, estrogen-responsive dermatoses, and hyperandro-genism in intact male dogs.

Nutritional Deficiency

Nutritional keratinization disorders that can cause ceruminous otitis are fatty acid deficiency, vitamin A–responsive dermatosis, and zinc-responsive dermatosis.

Fatty Acid Deficiency

Fatty acid binds water into the stratum corneum of normal skin, helping maintain the permeability properties of the skin barrier. Fatty acids also function as antioxidants.

Prolonged storage of dry dog and cat feed causes degradation of fatty acids, fatty acid deficiency, and reduced levels of antioxidants in animals that eat it. Animals fed home-cooked diets or reduced-fat diets may also have fatty acid deficiency. Gastrointestinal diseases that cause poor absorption result in fatty acid deficiency in spite of an adequate diet. In dogs, the essential fatty acids, linolenic acid and arachidonic acid, can be synthesized from linoleic acid. Cats lack the enzyme Δ-6-desaturase, and so they cannot convert linoleic acid to arachidonic acid. Therefore, cats require linolenic and arachidonic acids in their diets. Fatty acid deficiency in cats does not become clinically apparent until after many months of feeding a fatty acid–deficient diet.

Deficiency of fatty acids, especially arachidonic acid, in the diet may result in abnormalities in keratinization with microscopic epidermal changes (hypergranulosis, epidermal hyperplasia with orthokeratotic or parakeratotic hyperkeratosis).

Clinically, the animal with acute fatty acid deficiency has a dry, dull hair coat with generalized fine scaling of the skin. This also affects the ear, with the involvement of the pinnae and horizontal ear canal. In chronic conditions, there is epidermal thickening with concurrent greasiness of the ear pinnae and canal and the intertriginous and interdigital areas. The ceruminous otitis that accompanies this condition is made worse by secondary bacterial and *Malassezia* infections. Without appropriate treatment, pruritus and seborrhea become progressively worse.

Diagnosis and Treatment. Diagnosis of fatty acid deficiency is based on response to therapeutic levels of fatty acid supplementation. Making sure that an animal's diet contains the recommended amount of fat for proper health and that an animal on a reducing diet is given follow-up and routine veterinary care is mandatory. Commercially prepared and balanced veterinary omega-6 and omega-3 fatty acid supplementations are available. They contain linoleic, eicosapentaenoic, and docosahexaenoic acids. The latter two are marine lipids that modulate arachidonic acid metabolism, thus reducing inflammatory responses in the skin through prostaglandins and leukotrienes. They also mediate epidermal proliferation. The role of linoleic acid in controlling seborrheic dermatitis in dogs is well established. The proper storage of food at room temperature in airtight containers away from direct light is important to ensure that adequate levels of linoleic acid are present in the diet. Feeds should not be stored for prolonged periods.

Supplementation with sunflower, safflower, or vegetable oil at a dose of 5 mL per cup of dry or one can of dog food should elicit a response in 3 to 8 weeks. Similar results should be seen with commercially prepared veterinary supplements. Any secondary bacterial or *Malassezia* infection should also be treated.

Vitamin A–Responsive Dermatosis

Epithelial cells require vitamin A to maintain their integrity. Vitamin A is necessary for the proliferation and differentiation of keratinocytes. Cats lack the metabolic capability to convert carotene to vitamin A. The Cocker spaniel has a predisposition to this condition, which has also been reported in the Labrador retriever and miniature schnauzer.

Clinical Signs. The effects of vitamin A deficiency on the skin include marked hyperkeratosis of the epidermis, hair follicles, and sebaceous glands. The hyperkeratosis of the sebaceous glands results in blockage of the sebaceous secretion, giving rise to a papular-type skin eruption. In a generalized pattern, severe follicular plugging and hyperkeratotic plaques are usually secondarily infected with bacteria or *Malassezia* organisms. Ceruminous otitis is usually present, the severity of which depends on the chronicity of the condition. In most cases, a secondary bacterial or *Malassezia* infection is present.

Diagnosis and Treatment. The follicular changes present in dogs with vitamin A–responsive dermatosis and the histological finding of markedly disproportionate follicular orthokeratotic hyperkeratosis are enough to warrant treatment. The final diagnosis, however, depends on response to therapy. The condition responds to 400–800 IU/kg daily of Vitamin A orally once daily with a high-fat meal. Animals receiving such a high level of supplementation should be monitored for signs of toxicity.

Zinc-Responsive Dermatosis

Zinc-responsive dermatosis is a chronic keratinization disorder of dogs. Predilection for the disease is observed among the Alaskan malamutes and Siberian huskies, with a few reports in Doberman pinschers and Great Danes. There are two forms of this disorder: syndrome I and syndrome II.

Syndrome I. This syndrome affects mainly Siberian huskies and Alaskan malamutes, with reported cases in bull terriers. A genetic defect in the Alaskan malamute causes a diminished ability to absorb zinc from the gastrointestinal tract.

Despite a balanced diet, clinical signs usually appear in animals between 1 and 3 years of age. Clinical signs include alopecia with crusts and scales around the eyes and on the pinnae and horizontal canal of the ears. There is erythema with some form of erosion in these areas. Excessive sebum production and secondary bacterial and *Malassezia* infections are common; this condition is noticeable on the pinna of the ear and in the horizontal ear canal. Secondary bacterial and *Malassezia* infections of the ear canal cause the foul odor of the otitis present in this condition.

Syndrome II. Rapidly growing puppies fed diets either high in plant protein (phytate) or calcium or low or deficient in zinc have zinc-responsive dermatosis. Doberman pinschers, Labrador retrievers, Great Danes, standard poodles, and German shorthaired pointers are some of the breeds affected by this syndrome. Syndrome II may affect the ear canals in dogs, but hyperkeratotic plaques are the predominant lesions seen. Hyperkeratosis of the footpads and planum nasale are frequently present. Secondary bacterial infections are common.

Diagnosis. A thorough history, diet analysis, physical examination, and skin biopsy are important in the diagnosis of zinc-responsive dermatosis. Histological findings of hyperplastic superficial perivascular dermatitis with severe epidermal and follicular parakeratosis suggest the diagnosis.

Treatment. For dogs suffering from syndrome I, zinc supplementation is recommended (oral zinc sulfate or zinc methionine). For dogs with syndrome II, the correction of the diet usually produces a favorable response in 2 to 6 weeks. If dietary adjustment resolves the condition, there is no need for supplementation.

Allergic Dermatitis

Allergic dermatitis (see Chapter 7) in the dog and cat is a dermatological manifestation of the immune response elicited when an animal is exposed to allergens in the environment, food, insect saliva, or drugs. Allergic inhalant dermatitis (atopy), food hypersensitivity, and flea allergy dermatitis are the three most common hypersensitivity reactions in the dog and cat.

Allergic Inhalant Dermatitis (Atopy)

Allergic inhalant dermatitis (atopy) is a type I hypersensitivity reaction to environmental allergens seen in both dogs and cats. Predisposition to develop immunological reactions to allergen-specific immunoglobulin E (IgE) or IgG is inherited. Genetic predisposition for atopy exists in dogs, but not in cats.

Etiology and Pathogenesis. The causes of atopic dermatitis are various; they include weeds, grasses, tree pollens, molds, and other environmental products. The plethora of theories about the pathogenesis of atopy have in common the sensitization of animals to environmental allergens that results in a disease process.

Clinical signs are mediated by the degranulation of mast cells. When IgE fixed to mast cells reacts with specific allergens in the skin, the mast cells degranulate. When mast cells degranulate, they release vasoactive substances that cause vasodilation, edema, inflammation, smooth muscle contraction, and pruritus. Although the reaction occurs in cats, the exact pathogenesis of atopy in the cat is unknown.

Clinical Signs. Age of onset is between 1 and 3 years in the dog and between 6 and 24 months in the cat. The finding of otitis externa is often the only presenting sign of atopy in the dog. Other signs of atopy are foot licking and chewing, armpit and inguinal pruritus, face rubbing with conjunctivitis, focal to truncal alopecia depending on chronicity, secondary seborrhea, and secondary bacterial or *Malassezia* infections.

Otitis externa is rare in cats. Eosinophilic granuloma complex lesions and miliary dermatitis are the most common clinical manifestations of atopy in the cat. Cats also have head and neck pruritus of varying severity and self-induced alopecia. Chronic ceruminous otitis occurs in cases of atopy that either go untreated or fail to respond to therapy.

Diagnosis and Treatment. Identifying the offending allergens should be the focus of a diagnostic plan. However, history and physical examination are very important factors in the diagnosis of atopy. Every effort should be made to rule out parasitic diseases and food hypersensitivities before allergy testing is performed.

Both in vivo and in vitro allergy tests are available. The intradermal skin test (in vivo) is the most widely accepted test for atopy. The in vitro tests (radioallergosorbent test [RAST] and enzyme-linked immunosorbent assay [ELISA]) measure the level or concentration of allergen-specific IgG in the serum. The disadvantage of these tests is their high rate of false-positive reactions. They do not correlate well with intradermal skin tests. More clinicians are employing these tests, however, because of their ease of use. Nevertheless, the intradermal test is the most acceptable and preferred test for the diagnosis of atopy in the dog and cat.

The ceruminous otitis externa present in atopic dogs responds to therapy once the allergens are identified and hyposensitization is initiated. Topical and systemic therapies for the otitis should be considered in chronic cases. Therapy should be targeted to reduce inflammation and hypersecretion and hyperplasia of the ceruminous glands. Because most atopic dogs with ceruminous otitis have secondary bacterial or *Malassezia* infections, concurrent treatment of this condition is necessary to effect a good response. Avoiding offending allergens is the ideal treatment protocol for atopic dogs; when this is not possible, hyposensitization and other medical management should be initiated. Therapy in some animals is lifelong. Avoidance of the offending allergens, medical management of clinical signs, and hyposensitization are the keys to a successful management program for atopic animals.

Food Hypersensitivity

Food hypersensitivity is a type I, III, or IV hypersensitivity reaction. It is a nonseasonal, pruritic skin condition occurring in both dogs and cats. An affected animal may have received the same diet for years or may recently have been introduced to a new diet. Dogs and cats of any breed are susceptible.

Clinical Signs. Clinical signs of food allergy are variable. In the dog, there are atopy-like signs. Bilateral otitis externa, generalized pruritus, generalized secondary seborrhea, and signs resembling those of flea allergy dermatitis are common manifestations. Although gastrointestinal signs are uncommon, vomiting, diarrhea, and excessive flatulence may be present. In the cat, miliary dermatitis, pruritic head and neck dermatitis, eosinophilic granuloma complex lesions, and self-induced alopecia are common presentation signs.

Diagnosis and Treatment. History and physical examination play a major role in the diagnosis of food hypersensitivity. Food elimination diets, preferably with home-cooked food, is the best way to identify allergenic ingredients. If home cooking is not feasible, however, there are several commercially available hypoallergenic diets. The aims of a diet trial are to provide foods that the animal has had no previous exposure to, and to use diets that do not contain additives and preservatives. Because of the wide range of ingredients in commercially prepared diets, the best hypoallergenic diets are home cooked.

For proper diagnosis of food hypersensitivity, the recommended duration of a diet trial should be 10 to 13 weeks for dogs and 9 to 13 weeks for cats. Because animals with food allergy usually have concurrent atopy or flea allergy dermatitis, these conditions should be identified and treated before attempts are made to diagnose atopy. The proper management of food hypersensitivity consists of avoiding the offending allergenic foods and controlling clinical signs with topical or systemic medications.

Flea Allergy Dermatitis

Flea allergy dermatitis is the most common allergic dermatosis in the dog. The cutaneous reaction is due to the body's reaction to allergens present in the saliva of the flea. It can be a type I or type IV hypersensitivity reaction.

Clinical Signs. Pruritus, alopecia secondary to pruritus, and eruptions or papular crusts are most commonly present in the caudodorsal area of the body and often involve the dorsal tail area. Generalized cutaneous signs with secondary bacterial or *Malassezia* infections are usually present in chronic cases. Severe excoriations are present when pruritus is intense. Depending on the chronicity of the dermatitis, otitis externa can range from mild and hyperemic to ceruminous with severe epidermal hyperplasia. Pyotraumatic dermatitis and fibropruritic nodules may be present in chronic flea allergy dermatitis.

Diagnosis and Treatment. History, physical examination, identification of fleas and "flea dirt" with flea combing, and intradermal skin testing with flea allergens allow definitive diagnosis of flea allergy dermatitis. Response to therapy is most commonly used for definitive diagnosis of flea allergy dermatitis.

Various topical medications are available to kill both adult fleas and developing larval stages. Topical medications having residual effects for up to 1 month are now routinely used to kill adult fleas. Other products available have insect growth regulators and adulticides for pet, house, and yard treatments.

Concurrent bacterial infections should be treated, and medical management of pruritus, in the author's experience, significantly determines the response to antibacterial therapy.

Parasitic Dermatosis

Otodectes cyanotis

The most common parasite affecting the ear canal of dogs and cats, *Otodectes cyanotis* is transmitted by direct contact. Transmission among and between dogs and cats is extremely common. These ear mites are also present on other parts of the body. The sleeping habit of dogs and cats, in which the head is in close contact with the tail, makes the "tail-head region" a common site of infestation.

The adult mites live on the skin surface of the horizontal ear canal covered by a layer of debris. Mechanical irritation by mites causes the production of a waxy, brown cerumen. The ceruminous glands become dilated with cerumen. Epidermal scales and debris combine with cerumen to form a favorable medium for the growth of secondary bacteria and *Malassezia* species. Otic discharge complicated by secondary *Malassezia* or bacterial infection is usually malodorous, and patients are presented for the control of the odor rather than for symptoms of otitis. Secondary bacterial and *Malassezia* infections can mask the primary, underlying cause of the parasitic ceruminous otitis and thereby delay diagnosis.

Toxic and allergic substances produced by *Otodectes* mites cause hypersensitivity reactions in dogs and cats. The saliva of mites contains potent allergens that are responsible for this immune reaction. Ceruminous otitis externa can also be a result of *Otodectes* infestation.

Clinical Signs. Head shaking is common in animals with *Otodectes* infestation. The head shaking often leads to the formation of auricular hematomas. Intense pruritus of the ears is common, and animals can be presented with a noticeable head tilt, circling, and, sometimes in chronic untreated infestation, convulsions.

Otic examination may or may not reveal mites moving on hair shafts. An inflamed ear canal is not a hospitable environment for mites, so the migration of mites to other parts of the body is common. Ceruminous gland hyperplasia may make otic examination extremely difficult in patients with chronic *Otodectes* infestation. When there is hyperplasia of the ear canal, general anesthesia is recommended for otoscopic examination.

Histological findings include hyperplasia of the ceruminous glands in acute cases, along with epithelial parakeratosis and hyperplasia, an increase in inflammatory infiltrate, squamous metaplasia of apocrine ducts, and atrophy of hair follicles. Similar changes are present in chronic infections.

Diagnosis and Treatment. Diagnosis is by microscopic identification of the mites, determination of secondary bacterial or yeast identification, and response to treatment. The ears should be treated concurrently with the whole body. Various commercially prepared topical medications are available for the treatment of otic acariasis.

Sarcoptes scabiei

Although most commonly found on the pinnae of the ears, *Sarcoptes scabiei* mites can migrate into the external ear canal. The mechanical irritation and toxic substance produced by these mites lead to hyperproliferation of the ceruminous glands of the horizontal ear canal. Ceruminous otitis due to sarcoptic mites resolves once the primary problem and any secondary complications are treated.

Skin scrapings are not always positive for sarcoptic mites. If clinical signs and physical examination findings indicate sarcoptic infestation, it is best to treat the animal for the disorder and make a definitive diagnosis from the response to treatment.

Notoedres cati

The sarcoptic mite of cats, *Notoedres cati,* can also cause ceruminous otitis. Mechanical irritation in combination with the toxic substance and salivary antigens produced by the mites results in glandular irritation and proliferation.

Diagnosis and treatment are achieved by identifying the mite and implementing proper treatment. Sarcoptic mites are not always picked up on skin scrapings in the dog; in the cat, however, skin scrapings reveal numerous mites. Diagnosis is usually confirmed by response to treatment.

Otobius megnini

Otobius megnini, the spinous ear tick, has been implicated in ceruminous otitis of dogs and cats. Although this condition is rare, the larval and nymphal stages of this mite may feed on lymph and blood of the ear canal, resulting in irritation and subsequent hyperplasia of the ceruminous and sebaceous glands of the ear.

Diagnosis is made by identification of the larval or nymphal stages in the ear canal. Management of the tick population in the dog's environment is important to a successful treatment plan.

Mechanical removal of ticks with forceps is recommended. Grasping a tick on the head next to the animal's skin is ideal. Care should be taken not to rupture the tick, to prevent exposure to disease agents that may be present. Environmental treatment should be initiated and routinely maintained, especially in tick-infested areas.

Demodex canis

Some dogs with generalized demodicosis test positive for *Demodex canis* mite on ear swabs. Microscopic examination of ear swabs from these animals can be rewarding in the treatment and management of demodicosis. The mechanical irritation and irritation from toxins produced by these mites lead to the cystic dilation of the ceruminous glands of the ear. The result is hyperplasia of the ear canal in chronic conditions. The excessive cerumen produced by these glands is irritating and predisposes to secondary bacterial and *Malassezia* infections.

The treatment of generalized demodicosis with topical solution (amitraz) should involve instillation of the solution in the ear canal to achieve complete cure and prevent recurrence. When systemic medication is used, namely ivermectin or milbemycin oxime, treating the ear canal is not indicated. However, infected ears should be treated for secondary infections. The use of ivermectin and milbemycin oxime for the treatment of *Demodex* infestation is not approved by the FDA and its use is is extra-label (not approved for use in veterinary medicine for treating demodicosis).

Other Parasites

Other parasites responsible for ceruminous otitis are *Eutrombicula alfreddugési* and *Cheyletiella* species. Dermatophytes have also been implicated.

Tumors of the Ear Canal

Most tumors of the ceruminous glands are benign in the dog but malignant in the cat. Ceruminous and sebaceous gland adenomas, adenocarcinomas, basal cell carcinomas, fibrosarcomas, chondrosarcomas, trichoepitheliomas, mast cell tumors, ceruminous gland hyperplasia, and inflammatory polyps have been identified in the ears of dogs and cats. Nasopharyngeal polyps have been found in cats presented with otitis externa associated with ear masses. Tumors result in obstruction of the ear canal, and the most common tumors are of ceruminous gland origin. Ceruminous gland tumors are most frequently diagnosed in older male cats; these tumors have a high malignancy rate.

Ceruminous gland adenomas and carcinomas are the two most common tumors in the cat. The adenomas are smooth, nodular or pedunculated masses with intact epithelium. If there is secondary infection, the epithelium may be ulcerated.

Histologically, adenomas are differentiated cystic or tubular growths with cuboidal eosinophilic epithelium. Cystic contents are colloidal, orange to eosinophilic secretions. The mass present in the ear canal may invade the parotid salivary gland. Inflammatory polyps in dogs and cats may be misdiagnosed clinically as neoplasia. Histopathological diagnosis is necessary for differentiation of these masses.

Clinical Signs. Purulent, malodorous discharges are common clinical signs associated with any type of tumor in the ear canal. Secondary bacterial and *Malassezia* infections are common. Obstruction of the canal by these masses prevents drainage and results in the accumulation of debris and cerumen. The accumulation of this debris and cerumen irritates the epithelium of the canal, resulting in hyperplasia and hypersecretion of the ceruminous glands. Sinusitis and dysphagia are often present in cats with nasopharyngeal polyps

Diagnosis and Treatment. Otoscopic examination, preferably with the patient under general anesthesia, is necessary to determine the extent of these tumors. Although distinguishing between ceruminous gland hyperplasia and a neoplastic condition is difficult, it is important to determine the extent of the condition to plan for proper diagnostic procedures. For tumors of the ear, surgical intervention is the treatment of choice. Microscopic evaluation is necessary for a definitive diagnosis of tumors in the ear of dogs and cats.

Histological evidence of tumors (benign or malignant) warrants surgical intervention for tumor removal and proper ear drainage.

Environmental and Conformational Causes of Ceruminous Otitis

Moisture in the ear canal, due to high humidity, high ambient temperature, or improper drying of the ear after cleaning, and malodorous cerumen result in the absorption of an excessive amount of water by the epithelium of the ear canal. This leads to severe maceration of the ear canal with secondary infections. This condition is complicated by the poor ventilation observed in some dogs with pendulous pinnae. Covering of the external meatus by long pendulous ears prevents proper air circulation.

The improper use of ear medication, the use of harsh medications, and the inappropriate use of instruments in the ear cause irritation and abrasion, predisposing the ear canal to irritation and, subsequently, otitis externa with secondary infections and epithelial hyperplasia.

Properly drying the ears after cleaning, avoiding harsh medications, using appropriate instruments for ear cleaning, and performing routine otoscopic examination for early identification and treatment are mandatory for successful treatment of ceruminous otitis externa.

Suggested Readings

Griffin CE, Kwochka KW, MacDonald JM: Current Veterinary Dermatology: The Science and Art of Therapy. St. Louis, Mosby–Year Book, 1992.

Marino DJ, MacDonald JM, Matthiesen DT, et al: Results of surgery in cats with ceruminous gland adenocarcinoma. J Am Anim Hosp Assoc 30, 1994.

Nesbith GH, Ackerman LJ: Canine and feline dermatology: Diagnosis and treatment. Trenton, NJ, Veterinary Learning Systems, 1998.

Power HT, Ihrke PJ: Use of etretinate for treatment of primary keratinization disorders in Cocker spaniels. J Am Anim Hosp Assoc 201:419–429, 1992.

Scott DW, Miller WH, Griffin CE: Muller & Kirk's Small Animal Dermatology, 5th ed. Philadelphia, WB Saunders, 1995.

13

Advanced Imaging Techniques

Lisa J. Forrest, VMD, DACVR
(Radiology, Radiation Oncology)
Gregg Kortz, DVM, DACVIM (Neurology)

Computed Tomography

Computed tomography (CT) images are created by reconstruction of information obtained from an x-ray detector. The basic principle of CT is that a thin cross-section of the head can be examined from multiple angles with a pencil-like x-ray beam. The transmitted radiation is counted by a scintillation counter, fed into a computer for analysis, and reconstructed as a tomographic image. The images demonstrate a radiographic difference in the various soft tissues. The CT images can be adjusted to accentuate either the soft tissue or bony structures. CT excels in the detection of osseous changes, such as occurs in the osseous bulla in otitis media. With advances in CT scanners, images with spatial resolutions of less than 1 mm and differentiation of various soft tissues have become available.

CT findings are not specific for particular diseases but prove to be effective in demonstrating ongoing pathological processes. CT can be used to confirm the location and extent of a lesion and provide an anatomical site for diagnostic biopsy.

CT and magnetic resonance (MR) imaging are advanced imaging techniques useful in the evaluation of ear disease. CT and MR provide cross-sectional images that are exceptionally useful for evaluation of the complex anatomy of the skull. Most veterinary schools and many specialty practices have one or both of these imaging modalities either in-house or readily available through medical centers in which humans are treated. The goal of this chapter is to introduce these imaging modalities, in relation to ear disease, to the practicing veterinarian, veterinary student, and veterinary technician.

MR and CT have two main advantages over conventional radiography—images are tomographic (slices of the patient) and there is no superimposition of structures. MR is based on the properties of hydrogen protons in the presence of magnetic and radiofrequency fields and provides superior anatomic detail of soft tissue structures.

Despite the superior soft tissue detail obtained with MR, there are instances when CT is more desirable as an imaging modality. Due to the physical structure of bone, MR is not as useful as CT for cortical bone assessment. This limits its use in evaluation of tympanic bullae. Additionally, as noted by Chen and Pelizzari, artifacts due to magnetic field inhomogeneities may cause geometric distortion, limiting the accuracy of any measurement. Therefore, because structures are more geometrically precise on CT images, this is the preferred modality for computed radiotherapy planning.

According to Love et al., CT and radiographs have similar sensitivity for detection of otitis media. The sensitivity of disease detection using CT will most likely increase as equipment and image acquisition techniques improve. Due to the tomographic nature of CT and MR, detection of nasopharyngeal polyps is improved with these techniques. CT technology can display a larger gray scale than radiography, thereby enhancing contrast between structures. This allows viewing of images with both a soft tissue and a bone window by adjusting the gray scale on the monitor. Accurate detection of soft tissue changes and delineation of tumors and subtle bony lysis and proliferation are possible. However, radiography of tympanic bullae still remains a cost-effective screening tool for ear disease. The role of advanced imaging techniques is to define disease extent, precisely.

Case Discussion

Figure 13–1 shows CT images of a 5-year-old, neutered male Labrador retriever with a history of chronic bilateral ear infections over an 18-month period. Infections were somewhat responsive to antibiotics but recurred

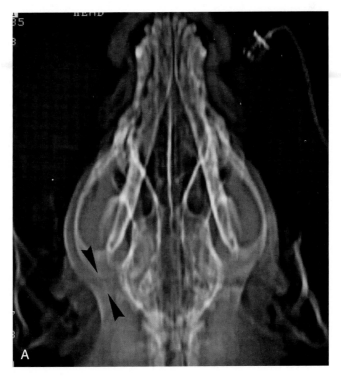

Figure 13–1

A, On the dorsoventral topogram of a Labrador retriever with chronic ear infection, the narrowed left ear canal *(arrowheads)* is visible.

Illustration continued on following page

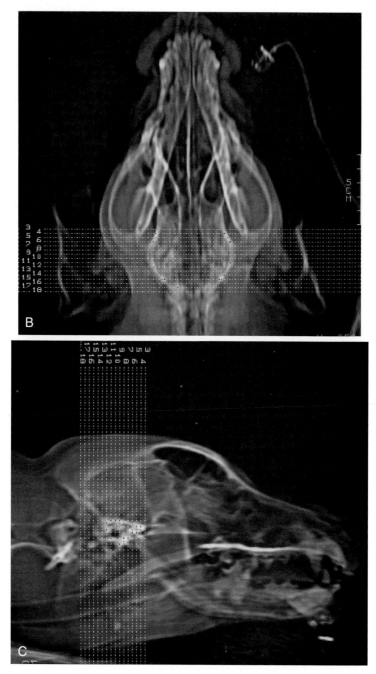

Figure 13–1 *Continued*

B, The topogram is used to select the anatomic area to be examined with the CT scanner. Dotted lines represent the location of each tomographic slice. *C,* CT imaging was confined to the tympanic bullae, as illustrated on the lateral topogram.

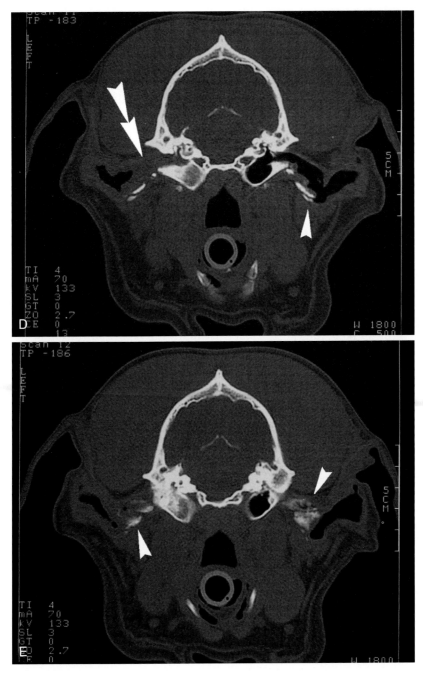

Figure 13–1 *Continued*

D, E, On transverse, tomographic images of the tympanic bullae bilateral otitis externa and left-sided otitis media can be seen. Note the stenotic left ear canal *(double arrowhead)* and mineralization of soft tissues of both ears *(small arrowheads),* indicating chronicity. Note the difference between the left and right tympanic bullae. The right bulla is air filled and normal. The left bulla is clearly abnormal with bony lysis and proliferation and filled with soft tissue material. Images *D* and *E* are adjacent slices, 3 mm thick, and are viewed with a bone window.

within 4 to 6 months. A CT scan of the skull was performed to accurately assess disease extent. On transverse, CT images (Fig. 13–1*D* and *E*) there is mineralization of both ear canals, osteomyelitis of the left bulla, and near-complete stenosis of the left ear canal by hyperplastic tissue. The right ear canal is patent. Upon completion of CT imaging, the ears were evaluated otoscopically, swabbed for culture and sensitivity, and irrigated. At that time, bilateral tympanic membrane rupture was noted. The final diagnosis was bilateral otitis externa and left otitis media secondary to *Pseudomonas* infection.

The therapeutic plan included the following regimen for a period of 6 to 8 weeks: dexamethasone/propylene glycol ear drops, oral ciprofloxacin, and enrofloxacin ear drops. The dog responded well to treatment, and at follow-up evaluation 4 weeks later, both tympanic membranes had regrown. Long-term therapy of ear cleaning and medication to prevent clinical *Pseudomonas* recurrence was instituted.

Figure 13–2 is transverse CT images of a 14-year-old, neutered female Birman cat with a biopsy-confirmed diagnosis of squamous cell carcinoma of the left tympanum. The CT scan was performed to define tumor extent and for computed radiotherapy planning before initiation of treatment. Computed treatment planning improves treatment accuracy and provides a more uniform dose distribution within the tumor volume. Although bony lysis was noted on skull radiographs, the tumor extent was more defined and easier to delineate on CT images.

As can be seen on the CT scan, the gross tumor burden was quite extensive in this cat. Therapy goals were palliative rather than curative due to severity of disease. The cat initially responded to radiotherapy and chemotherapy with partial resolution of the physical abnormalities secondary to the tumor. One month after completion of radiotherapy there was evidence of tumor progression and worsening of the left head tilt (presenting complaint). The cat became anorexic and the owner elected euthanasia.

These two case examples demonstrate the utility of CT images in the evaluation and treatment of ear disease in companion animals. With advanced imaging techniques such as CT and MR, precise definition of disease extent is possible. Tomographic images provide important information that is essential to medical, surgical, and radiotherapy planning.

Magnetic Resonance Imaging

MR is a noninvasive procedure that does not involve ionizing radiation. It involves imaging of the proton, the positively charged spinning nucleus of hydrogen atoms that are abundant in tissues containing water, proteins, lipids, and other macromolecules. Because of its spin and charge, a proton

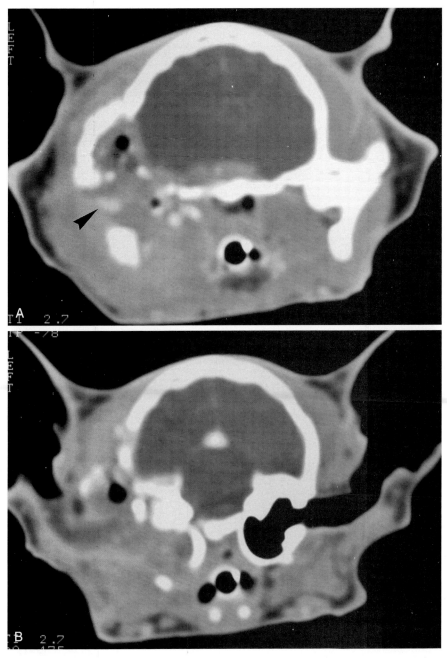

Figure 13–2

A, Transverse, contrast-enhanced tomographic image at the level of the temporomandibular joint of a cat with squamous cell carcinoma of the left tympanum. Note the bony destruction of the left side of the skull and contrast enhancement of the mass *(arrowhead). B, C,* On transverse images, that are 9 and 18 mm caudal to the temporomandibular joint, respectively; there is complete destruction of the left bulla and obliteration of the external ear canal.

Illustration continued on following page

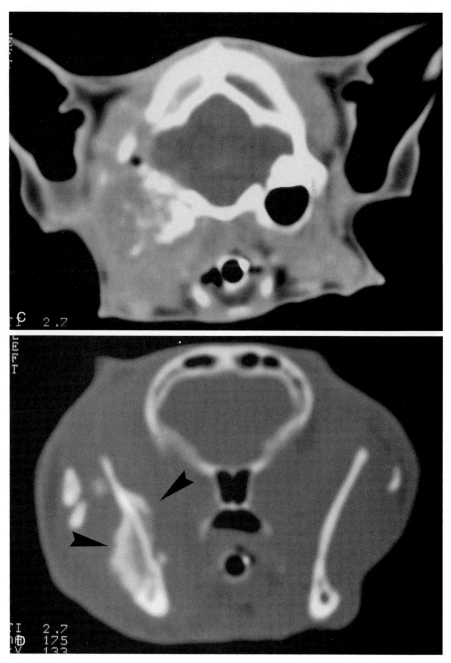

Figure 13–2 *Continued*

Figure 13–2 *A–C* is viewed with a soft tissue window. *D,* Transverse tomographic image, viewed with a bone window, is 12 mm rostral to the temporomandibular joint. Note the aggressive bony remodeling of the left mandibular ramus *(arrowheads)* secondary to tumor invasion.

has a minute magnetic field. When radiofrequency energy at the appropriate frequency, called the Larmor frequency, is applied, protons aligned with the magnetic field absorb energy and reverse their direction. The protons subsequently release the absorbed energy and "relax" back to the original alignment at a rate determined by the T1 and T2 relaxation times. The relaxation times depend on the physical and chemical characteristics of the tissue. Images can be T1-, T2-, or proton density–weighted. The degree of weighting depends on the pulse sequence, repetition time, and echo time chosen.

Because variation in T1 and T2 values are so much greater than variations in tissue density, MR provides better soft tissue contrast than does CT. MR is also superior to CT in detection of pathological tissue features such as edema, cysts, vascularity, hemorrhage, and necrosis. The multiplanar imaging capability of MR permits better definition of anatomical relationships.

Gadolinium-enhanced T1-weighted images are preferred for the diagnosis of intracranial neoplasia in humans. They are more sensitive than double-dose contrast-enhanced CT images.

MR is very sensitive for localizing central nervous system inflammatory disorders. For example, diseases resulting in demyelination can cause a decrease in the lipid content of myelin and an increase in the water content, therefore increasing the signal intensity on T2-weighted images. Image patterns may be characteristic for some diseases, but as with CT, a microscopic diagnosis is still required.

Case Discussion

The images in Figure 13–3A and B are from a 17-year-old, spayed female domestic shorthair cat. The presenting complaint was a progressive 3-month history of a left head tilt, mild ataxia involving all limbs, and difficulty swallowing food. Past drug therapy included several different antibiotics with no apparent clinical improvement. Squamous cell carcinoma was the histological diagnosis of the osseous bulla and surrounding soft tissues.

The images in Figure 13–4A–D are from an 8-month-old male Persian. The presenting complaint was a 2-week history of a discharge from the right ear canal and an acute onset of a right cerebellar-vestibular syndrome. This was an example of a bacterial otitis externa, media/interna with extension through the petrous temporal bone and central nervous system involvement.

The images in Figure 13–5A–D are from a 4-year-old, neutered male domestic long hair. The presenting complaint was a 2- to 3-month history of a chronic ear discharge from the left ear canal and progressive neurological deficits. This case was an example of a bacterial otitis externa, media/interna with extension through the petrous temporal bone and

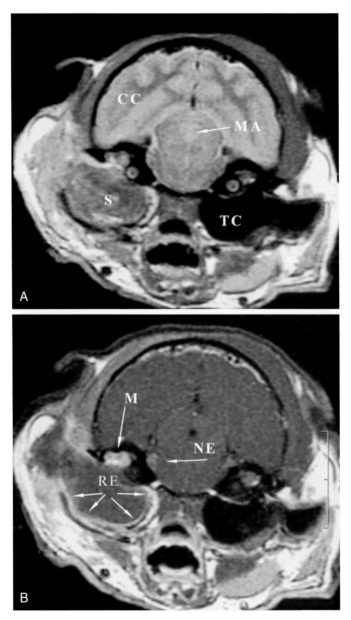

Figure 13-3

A, A 3-mm thickness proton-weighted transverse image at the level of the tympanic cavity in a female domestic shorthair. A soft tissue mass is identified within the left tympanic cavity. (CC, cerebral cortex; MA, mesencephalic aqueduct; TC, tympanic cavity; S, soft tissue mass.) *B,* A 3-mm thickness postcontrast T1-weighted transverse image at the same level as image *A.* The soft tissue mass has a contrast-enhancing rim and smaller homogeneous contrast-enhancing component with extension to the adjacent neural tissue. (RE, contrast-enhancing rim; M, contrast-enhancing mass; NE, contrast-enhancing neural tissue.)

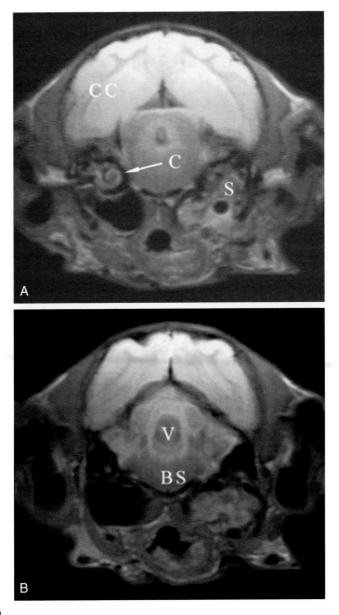

Figure 13–4

A, A 3-mm thickness proton-weighted transverse image at the level of the tympanic cavity in a male Persian. A complex soft tissue mass with different single intensities is identified within the right tympanic cavity. (CC, cerebral cortex; C, cochlea; S, soft tissue mass.) *B,* A 3-mm thickness proton-weighted transverse image at 0.5 mm caudal to image *A.* (BS, brain stem; V, dilated fourth ventricle.)

Illustration continued on following page

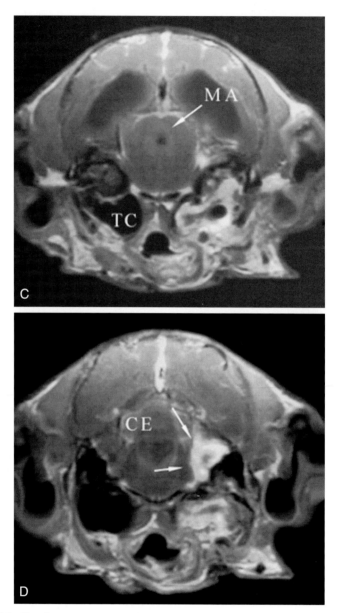

Figure 13–4 *Continued*

C, A 3-mm thickness postcontrast T1-weighted transverse image at the level of image *A.* Heterogeneous contrast enhancement of the complex mass is identified. (MA, mesencephalic aqueduct; TC, tympanic cavity.) *D,* A 3-mm thickness postcontrast T1-weighted transverse image at the level of image *B.* Contrast enhancement of the adjacent cerebellum and brain stem is identified. (*Arrows,* contrast enhancement; CE, cerebellum.)

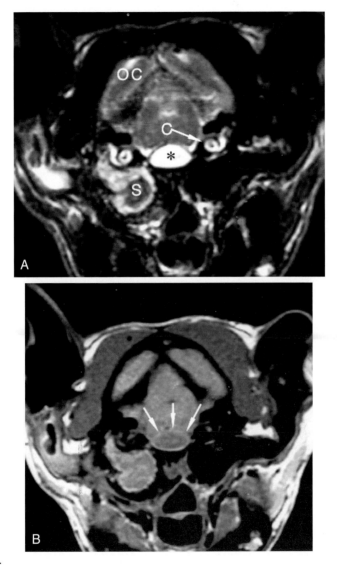

Figure 13–5

A, A 3-mm thickness T2-weighted transverse image at the level of the tympanic cavity in a male domestic short hair. A complex soft tissue mass with different single intensities is identified within the left tympanic cavity. An additional area of high signal intensity is identified ventral to the brain stem. (OC, occipital cortex; C, cochlea; S, soft tissue mass,* high signal intensity area.) *B,* A 3-mm thickness proton-weighted transverse image at the level of image *A.* (* - rim of high signal intensity.)

Illustration continued on following page

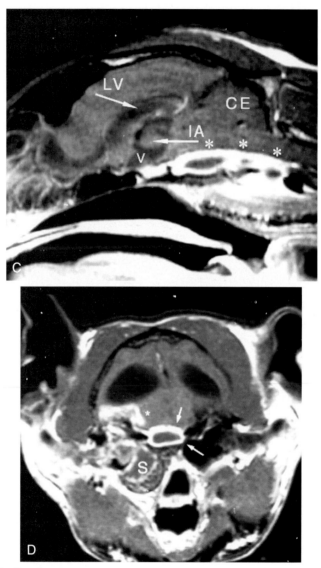

Figure 13–5 *Continued*

C, A 3-mm thickness postcontrast T1-weighted sagittal image. Contrast-enhancing mass ventral to the brain stem is identified. (LV, lateral ventricle; V, third ventricle; CE, cerebellum; IA, interthalamic adhesion,* contrast-enhancing mass.) *D,* A 3-mm thickness postcontrast T1-weighted transverse image 0.5 mm caudal to image A. Heterogeneous contrast enhancement of the soft tissue mass within the left tympanic cavity is identified. In addition, the area ventral to the brain stem demonstrates a rim of contrast enhancement with adjacent cerebral contrast enhancement noted as well. (S, soft tissue mass; *arrows,* rim of contrast enhancement,* adjacent cerebral enhancement.)

central nervous system involvement with abscess formation ventral to the brain stem.

In conclusion, MR offers many advantages over CT: superior tissue contrast, the ability to obtain images in multiple planes, the absence of artifacts caused by bone, vascular imaging capability, and the absence of ionizing radiation. The disadvantage of MR is a longer scanning time, which makes MR more sensitive to motion artifacts. The clinician should recognize the advantages and disadvantages of each modality and request the procedure that will give the required information with the least risk to the patient.

Suggested Readings

Barthez PY, Koblik PD, Hornof WJ, et al: Apparent wall thickening in fluid filled versus air filled tympanic bulla in computed tomography. Vet Radiol Ultrasound 37:95–98, 1996.

Chen GTY, Pelizzari CA: Imaging in radiotherapy. *In* Khan FM, Potish RA (eds): Treatment Planning in Radiation Oncology, Baltimore, Williams & Wilkins, 1998, pp 11–31.

Love NE, Kramer RW, Spodnick GJ, et al: Radiographic and computed tomographic evaluation of otitis media in the dog. Vet Radiol Ultrasound 36:375–379, 1995.

Seitz SE, Lasonsky JM, Marretta SM: Computed tomographic appearance of inflammatory polyps in three cats. Vet Radiol Ultrasound 37:99–104, 1996.

14

Diagnosis and Treatment of Pruritic Otitis

Steven A. Melman, VMD

M ost cases of acute otitis externa are pruritic. The pet is presented to the veterinarian for scratching at the ear, erythematous pinnae, shaking of the head, or apparent pain when the ears are manipulated. The differential diagnosis for pruritus is extensive and is dealt with in textbooks on dermatology.

This chapter entails a "rapid-fire" clinical trial approach to the treatment of pruritus in a pet with or without otitis externa. Such an approach addresses treatment for several different causes of pruritus at once. This regimen not only promises the best chance to achieve fast and lasting relief from pruritus but also allows the veterinarian to make a rapid clinical diagnosis based on the response to the various elements involved in the trial. The chapter concludes with a program of treatment for otitis.

Perhaps the most common cause of acute otitis externa is hypersensitivity. The most common hypersensitivities encountered in small animal practice are flea allergy, food allergy, and atopy. Dogs with atopic dermatitis are presented to the veterinarian with a clinical history of pruritus of the feet, face, axilla, and ears. It has been estimated that as many as 70% of dogs with atopy have otitis externa and pruritic ears. In dogs and cats with food hypersensitivity, otic pruritus may be the only sign of disease. Flea allergy may contribute to overall pruritus but rarely causes otic pruritus by itself.

If the clinician suspects atopy, a pretreatment blood sample for in vitro allergy testing should be obtained prior to the start of this pruritic clinical trial, which involves the use of some corticosteroids. The blood should be spun and the serum frozen. Frozen serum can be submitted for in vitro allergy testing as long as 60 to 90 days after sampling without affecting the results. Testing and therapy for atopy are both tedious and expensive; the treatment is lifelong. The clinical trial described here may provide the client proof that the pet is suffering from hypersensitivity, making the client's decision to proceed with testing and hyposensitization easier.

Of course, a good physical examination and observational skills are not to be neglected in the attempt to sort out the etiology of dermatologic disease. It is prudent to perform skin scraping and analysis, fecal analysis, heartworm testing, fungal culture, skin and ear cytological evaluations, and other tests as indicated by clinical common sense during the initial examination.

In addition, recheck visits and the observational skills of the client are crucial to securing an accurate diagnosis. The veterinarian should have the client keep a daily diary of the pet's response, using a scale of 1 through 10 to quantify the intensity of pruritus, erythema, pain, any discharge from the ear, and head shaking.

Clinical Treatment Trial for Pruritus

This clinical trial for pruritus should be performed in conjunction with topical ear treatment (see later). Start all actions on Day 1.

Step 1: Shampoo Therapy

Of the estimated 116 million dogs and cats in the United States, 12% to 20% have allergy-induced skin problems that require frequent bathing, preferably with "hypoallergenic" shampoos.

Shampoo therapy has moved to the forefront in the treatment of all but the rarest skin disorders. It involves the use of cleansing, moisturizing, antiseborrheic, degreasing, antiparasitic, antibacterial, antifungal, and antipruritic shampoos. Specific products and protocols usually are selected on the basis of the presenting morphological characteristics, such as dryness, oiliness, scaling, inflammation, and associated pyoderma. Generally, the use of a milder, more elegant product before a coarser, more potent one increases the pet owner's compliance with the regimen and reduces the risk of side effects, such as irritation.

Various issues must be considered in the selection of therapeutic shampoos to relieve pets' specific symptoms.

Cleansers and Moisturizers

Cleansing and moisturizing shampoos are designed to do just what their names imply. The mechanical process of bathing (even with water alone) helps remove scales, crusts, organisms, dander, loose hair, and other debris. All such shampoos should be pH-adjusted for dogs, which have the highest skin pH of any mammal (6.2 to 7.2), including humans.

Oils and Conditioners

Moisturizing agents, such as bath oils, conditioners, emollients, and humectants, may be applied after bathing and rinsing to soften, lubricate, and rehydrate the skin. They can be used on a more regular basis for dryness.

Antiseborrheic Treatments

Seborrhea is the term used for any skin disease involving dry *(sicca)* or greasy *(oleosa)* scaling. The term also encompasses disorders in the formation of keratin, a complex protein unique to the skin, hair follicles, and nails. Today, many experts prefer the term *disorders of keratinization*. This subject is covered in detail elsewhere in this book.

The epidermis is completely replaced every 22 days in the normal dog. Epidermal cell turnover time in dogs suffering from idiopathic seborrhea, which is more common among Cocker spaniels, may be as short as 3 to 6 days. This fast turnover creates a defect in the normal protective barrier, which may result in dry or greasy scales, comedones, alopecia, inflammation, crusts, pyoderma, and pruritus. Any of these conditions, in turn, may lead to further skin damage. In these cases, it is important to slow the turnover process and treat the secondary problems.

Bathing Procedure

Bathe the pet daily in a hypoallergenic shampoo. If the pet remains itchy after these baths, an oatmeal shampoo or conditioner may help resolve mild pruritus. If pyoderma, *Malassezia* dermatitis, or seborrhea oleosa is present, degreasing and antiseptic shampoo should be used every 2 to 3 days. The author prefers a shampoo with acetic acid and boric acid (MalAcetic, DermaPet) followed by an acetic acid–boric acid conditioner. This unique combination kills bacteria and yeasts on the skin.

Shampoo therapy should be used as a component of the clinical trial for 3 weeks. If the pet improves symptomatically, the owner should continue the bathing.

Step 2: Fatty Acid Diet Supplementation

Supplementing the pet's diet with an omega-3/6 fatty acid supplement should reduce the inflammation associated with pruritus. Antioxidants such as vitamin E and vitamin C should be included in the supplement because they are depleted more rapidly when there is fish oil (omega-3) in the diet. In some breeds, zinc is also a useful supplement when a zinc-responsive dermatosis is present.

Step 3: Food Elimination Diet

Conduct a strict food elimination diet for a minimum of 21 days; in some food-allergic dogs, 60 to 90 days may be required to show beneficial effect. Many diets that can be used for the food elimination trial are commercially available. They contain either uncommon, novel protein sources (venison, rabbit, duck, fish) or purified low-molecular-weight polypeptides. The author prefers to use a home-cooked vegetarian diet (see the box).

PREPARATION AND USE OF ALL-VEGETABLE HYPOALLERGENIC DIET*

1. Vegetable puree (multiple batch)

    Three undrained #1 cans of:
        carrots, peas, green beans, and tomatoes, and greens (kale, dock, spinach, or mustard)
    One 10 oz. package of chopped frozen broccoli

    Boil the broccoli in 2 cups of water until tender. Combine with the other vegetables in a large kettle, mix and puree until smooth. Fill 18 one-pint plastic containers and freeze.

2. Rice (prepare as required)

    2½ cups rice
    5 cups water
    ½ cup sunflower oil
    1 tsp salt

    Mix ingredients, bring to boil, reduce heat, and simmer until water is absorbed. Allow to cool.

3. Thaw 1 pint of vegetable puree and add to rice; mix thoroughly.

4. Feed ½–¾ cup per 10 lbs body weight twice daily. Monitor weight weekly. Do not add meat supplements.

*Modified from Byrne K: Food allergy. *In* Skin Diseases of Dogs and Cats, Potomac, MD, DermaPet, Inc, 1994.

Step 4: Corticosteroids

Administer a low-dose corticosteroid for 12 days (e.g., prednisone at 0.5 mg/lb bid). Use a tapering dosage regimen that ends with 0.5 mg per pound every other day. The rationale is to break the pruritic cycle and to observe whether the pruritus is responsive to corticosteroids.

Step 5: Treatment for Infections

If the pet has pyoderma, use an antibiotic such as cephalexin at 10–15 mg per pound bid for a minimum of 21 days. If the ear is also infected with bacteria, prescribe a fluoroquinolone such as enrofloxacin at 5 mg/lb bid or 10 mg/lb once daily.

If *Malassezia* dermatitis is present, bathing with the acetic acid–boric acid shampoo as described in step 1 and antibiotic therapy will usually control the pruritus. On rare occasions, or when there is very deep involvement of the skin with *Malassezia,* oral ketoconazole at 10 mg/kg once daily or itraconazole at 5 mg/kg once daily may be used. Duration of treatment varies, but should be at least 2 weeks.

Treatment for Infestations

Treat scabies, other ectoparasites, and some endoparasites with a trial of ivermectin. In all breeds except collies or their mixes, use ivermectin (Bovine Ivomec, MSD/AgVet) at 0.1 mL/10 lb body weight given subcutaneously. Use every 7 to 10 days for 4 treatments. The extra-label use of this drug requires informed consent of the client.

Endoparasite Therapy

Treat phantom endoparasites with a dewormer that kills whipworms.

Flea Control

If not already on flea control, begin flea control program.

Analyzing the Results of the Trial

If the clinical signs stop while the prednisone and ivermectin are being given and never return, the diagnosis is ectoparasites, most likely scabies, or ear mite hypersensitivity: The ivermectin killed the parasites, and the prednisone reduced the pruritus.

If the response is more gradual and the pruritus does not return after bathing with the acetic acid–boric acid shampoo and/or ketoconazole or itraconazole, cutaneous *Malassezia* infection is the likely cause. Unfortunately, *Malassezia* infection is often a secondary complication that perpetuates otic pruritus in many atopic dogs. An acetic acid–boric acid ear cleaner may need to be used on a maintenance basis once or twice a week to control otic *Malassezia* yeasts.

If the pruritus returns between day 12 and day 21, a cortisone-responsive hypersensitivity is most likely, and allergy testing should be done. The frozen pretreatment serum sample can then be submitted for in vitro allergy testing.

If itching remains controlled comfortably after the original pretreatment diet is re-instituted, the possibility that the animal has a fatty acid or shampoo therapy–responsive atopy is high. Primary food allergy should be suspected if the itching returns within 72 hours after the hypoallergenic diet is withdrawn and the pet is returned to the pretreatment diet.

Bacterial hypersensitivity may be suspected if the itching returns within 30 days after the antibiotic is stopped, provided that the pruritus was controlled during antibiotic therapy. If the itching disappears after a second course of antibiotic therapy, the diagnosis is confirmed.

Keratinization disorders, including hypothyroidism, skin neoplasia, and other less common primary skin diseases, prevent the itch from fully resolving. Incomplete treatment of *Malassezia* dermatitis or the failure to treat all contact animals for scabies may cause persistent pruritus. Biopsy of the skin may be helpful in many circumstances to identify the etiology of pruritic skin diseases.

In many cases of acute otitis externa without progressive pathological changes, resolution of pruritic skin disease also decreases otic pruritus. However, the skin of the ear is treated differently from the skin of the trunk, primarily with concentrated topical medications.

Ear Therapy

The following is a simple, logical, progressive method of providing ear therapy. Prior to initiating these steps, appropriate specimens for cytological evaluation or culture should be obtained. The clinician should perform the steps in the order given (no skipping); if one step does not resolve the problem, therapy should continue to the next step if necessary.

Step 1: Ear Cleaning

Clean the ear thoroughly using a nonototoxic ear cleaner in the hospital so that a thorough otic examination can be performed, including assessment of the tympanic membrane. The author prefers an acetic acid–boric acid ear cleaner. Problems may arise when detergents and alcohols are used as an ear cleaner in an ear in which the eardrum may be ruptured. Use anesthesia when appropriate.

Acetic acid and boric acids in combination have been shown to be an effective combination in vivo to treat *Malassezia* otitis (Gotthelf, 1997). In many cases, continued daily ear cleansing by the owner at home for 1 week is all that is needed. Twice-weekly maintenance cleaning may prevent recurrence of *Malassezia* infection. Cleaning the ear is important in removing surface debris from the affected ear canal epithelium. Apply medications, if needed, after cleaning.

Procedure

1. Apply approximately 5 mL (1 tsp) of the ear cleaner into the ear canal, and massage thoroughly. A cotton ball may be inserted into the canal to protect against drenching if the pet shakes its head.

2. For maximum benefit, allow the ear cleaner to remain in the ear canal for at least 5 minutes before attempting to manually clean it.

3. Clean the ear by using a cotton ball at the opening of the ear canal to absorb liquid and debris that has been dislodged. With each day of treatment, less debris will be removed.

4. Stop daily cleaning when the cotton ball remains free of debris after cleaning.

In dry or irritated ears with little debris and wax, the cotton ball may be irritating. In these cases, a tiny bulb syringe or Water Pik can be helpful. Warmed solutions seem to soften waxy debris. In problem ears, the frequency of cleaning may need to be increased to one to three times daily.

It is important to remember that infected ears are very acidic, a condition that inactivates some antibiotics commonly used in the ear, such as gentamicin and amikacin. Many ear cleaners are also acidic. Waiting 30 minutes after cleaning to apply these antibiotics may be warranted.

Cleaning with EDTA-tris

One nonototoxic alkalinizing agent that the literature reports to have primary antimicrobial properties is ethylenediaminetetraacetic acid with tris (EDTA-tris [TrizEDTA, DermaPet]). Follow the preceding instructions on how to clean an ear, substituting the alkalinizing EDTA-tris for the acidic ear cleaner. It appears that pretreatment with this agent increases the antimicrobial activity of many antibiotics used to treat ear disease. It is especially useful in stubborn cases of *Pseudomonas* otitis. Gentamicin or enrofloxacin may be added to the EDTA-tris solution.

Step 2: Topical Therapy

Logical otic therapy is based on the results of otic examination and cytological evaluation. In bacterial infections, antibiotics should be used. In yeast infection, use an anti-yeast therapy. In inflammation (neutrophils on the cytological specimen) or erythema, use a topical corticosteroid. If ear mites are present, use a topical insecticide or topical ivermectin. After the ear has been cleaned, apply the topical formula (see details in box).

TOPICAL EAR FORMULA

12 mL acetic acid–boric acid ear cleaner

2 mL enrofloxacin injectable

6 mg dexamethasone sodium phosphate (for greater solubility)

Also add as appropriate:

0.5–1 mL medical-grade dimethyl sulfoxide (DMSO)

0.5 mL ivermectin

Step 3: Systemic Therapy

Steps 3a and 3b may be performed separately or concurrently. They are the logical next steps after ear cleaning and use of a topical formula fail to cause remission of disease. Steps 1 and 2 are continued, and Step 3a and/or 3b is added.

Step 3a: Begin use of a systemic antibiotic, such as a fluoroquinolone (Baytril, Bayer), at double the recommended dose.

Step 3b: If inflammation or purulent material is present, use a short-acting systemic corticosteroid.

Step 4: Further Complications

When steps 1 through 3 do not cause remission of disease after 2 weeks, re-examine the ears. For stenosis and strangulation of the canal, use a 1.5-inch, 20-gauge needle to inject approximately 0.5 mL methylprednisolone acetate (Depo-Medrol) between the epithelium and cartilage as distally in the canal as possible.

If the eardrum is bulging, a myringotomy may be performed to relieve the pressure and pain and allow collection of a culture specimen from the middle ear. If the eardrum is ruptured, infuse a combination of 1–2 mg dexamethasone sodium phosphate and 10–20 mg enrofloxacin directly into the tympanic bulla.

The use of corticosteroids is multifunctional. Although we are most familiar with the anti-inflammatory properties of such agents, their ability to reduce viscosity of the secretions and exudate is a noteworthy goal in cases of otitis media.

Step 5: Step 4 and Culture and Sensitivity Testing

Many dermatologists recommend a culture specimen from each ear in difficult cases to assess the bacterial microflora. It is possible for a pet to have different bacteria in each ear and for otitis media to be complicated by bacteria that are not normally found in the external ear. Topical treatment with antibiotics achieves much higher tissue levels than the minimum inhibitory concentration (MIC) reported by the laboratory, so bacteria resistant according to culture results may be susceptible to higher topical doses of the same drug.

Step 6: EDTA-tris

In stubborn bacterial otitis externa or otitis media, use EDTA-tris (TrizEDTA) prior to the instillation of the antimicrobial. Clean the ear thoroughly for 7 to 21 days. EDTA-tris is an alkaline solution with a pH of 8.0. There are reports in the literature that this agent has primary microbiocidal properties, particularly against *Pseudomonas*. There is also evidence that EDTA-tris potentiates the action of antibiotics that are inactivated by other acidifying ear cleansers. If *Pseudomonas* is suspected from cytological evaluation or found by culture, use the appropriate systemic and topical antibiotics after 15-minute pretreatments with EDTA-tris.

Step 7: Surgery

If (1) corticosteroid injection into the ear canal epithelium fails to open up an inflamed, swollen, occluded ear canal (Step 4), (2) permanent pathological changes are evident, or (3) there is severe calcification of the ear canal, surgery of the ear canal is indicated for relief of pain and to allow for drainage.

Reference

Gotthelf L, Young S: A new treatment for canine otitis externa. Vet Forum 14(8):46–53, 1997.

15

Marketing Ear Care and Otitis Therapy: The Nuts and Bolts

Ronald E. Whitford, DVM

The veterinary profession is currently undergoing major changes in its relationship with today's pet owners. Over the past several years, new products introduced and distributed only through licensed veterinarians have led many practices to become more vendor-oriented than service-oriented. Now, with the possibility that many of these products will be available over the counter, the savvy practice owner has reason to worry about future income potential.

From a profit perspective, it is better to select potential profit centers that offer minimal competition from other sources. Placing the emphasis on providing professional services rather than selling products has the potential to be much more successful because of the limited competition. The marketing of professional services rather than products also has the advantage of a much higher gross profit margin because the income generated from providing a service requires a much lower "hard cost" in materials and supplies used.

The only true additional costs of providing additional services would be the hard costs of the materials needed to provide those services. In most cases, the support personnel, the facility, the utilities, and other categories of daily overhead operating costs do not change significantly, thereby making diversification of the practice through providing additional services very cost-effective while also having the potential to enhance the practice's actual net income.

First the bad news: Latest surveys show that the pet populations are stable. Because the number of veterinarians entering practice continues to rise, one would assume that the number of pets seen by each veterinarian will decrease. Therefore, it is important not to lose the pets currently seen in a practice. It is well-known that the average practice loses 30% of its clients a year from normal attrition—owners moving, pets dying, and so on. With pet populations remaining stable, it is therefore necessary for the veterinarian to recommend and to be able to provide all the services needed by the limited number of pets seen on a daily basis.

Now the good news: Pets are predisposed to many conditions because of a specific breed predilection or their environment. This is especially true for ear diseases. Pets are no longer considered disposable. The human-pet bond is known to be strengthening. People want the same high quality of care for their pets as they want for themselves. There are now more than 6 million dogs and 6 million cats in the United States more than 6 years old. As pets age, many become more bonded as loved family members. Also, the aging process involves many medical problems, including ear problems. Ear care programs can therefore be developed to catch these problems early or even to prevent them. Also, the U.S. economy is good, providing many clients with more potential income to spend on their four-legged family members.

Of all the marketing options we veterinarians have today, none is more professional or more restricted to our use than that of professional mar-

keting of services related to ear care. These services are not easily duplicated by other sources because of the expertise required to diagnose and treat the various ear conditions. The services will be accepted by a veterinarian's best clients: those who regard their pets as family members. Buyers of these services cannot readily compare prices for them, so the services tend to have a higher gross margin markup percentage, resulting in greater profitability. A survey of veterinary practices today would show that only a small percentage of practices currently place significant emphasis on ear care as a major profit center.

Other reasons for a veterinarian to put emphasis on ear care are as follows:

- Pets have two ears, thereby providing more chances of finding problems.
- The ear canals of dogs and cats are formed anatomically in such a way as to increase the potential for problems.
- People do not put a price on pain control. Ear infections often hurt—and the pain is perceived by the owner who observes the pet scratching, shaking its head, or whining when the ears are touched.
- Ear infections are likely to be lifelong problems. (A major reason for chronic otitis is the failure to recognize allergies as the underlying cause.) Failure of the client to return for recheck and employing too short a treatment time contribute to ineffective ear treatment. It is just human nature for many clients not to return when requested, so the condition surfaces again and again.
- People often feel guilty when their pet has a recurrence once they understand that it has occurred because of their failure to continue the treatment. The feeling of guilt makes the client more willing to seek more extensive treatments at a later time.
- Clients often leave one veterinarian for another because the first veterinarian failed to adequately treat their pet's ear infection.

What is Marketing, Anyway?

Marketing is nothing more than communication. It is simply providing sufficient facts and benefits about the services we offer in such a way as to make the client *want* to accept our recommendations. To do this, we must *believe* that the services we provide are beneficial to both the client and the pet. We must first know what we offer—the facts and benefits of the services we can provide. We must also take time to understand our clients, learning the particular "hot buttons" for each one.

Some marketing fundamentals to remember:

1. Be prepared. You must know the why and what as well as the "how" for the services and products you recommend.

2. Avoid giving the impression of high-pressure selling. Clients love to buy but hate to "be sold." Few people buy from pushy sales personnel, at least not more than once.

3. Marketing is not manipulative or unethical; it is simply providing facts and benefits.

4. Clients must first trust us and have confidence in us as doctors rather than as just vendors.

5. We must discover the needs of each client in order to sell a solution. The key is helping the client find the right solution to the specific problem.

6. Clients must believe we care. We must make a friend before we can make a sale. It is still true that *people don't care how much you know until they know how much you care.* We show we care by being sincerely interested, listening, asking good questions, and knowing what to recommend by interpreting what the client wants along with what the pet needs.

A lot of research has been conducted on the buying process. People buy to feel better or to solve a problem. They purchase veterinary services (1) to make their pet feel better, which in turn makes them feel better, or (2) to solve a problem with the pet, which again makes them feel better. Eighty per cent of all purchases are based on emotions rather than logic. Therefore, it is important to first determine the emotional needs of the client. *Emotional buying requires emotional selling.* Marketing is nothing more than a battle of perceptions. We must position ourselves as caring, concerned health professionals interested in providing the best that veterinary medicine has to offer.

Clients must first trust us before they will accept our recommendations. Some principles important to understand are:

- People are interested in themselves and want to be noticed.
- People crave to feel important and be appreciated.
- People want to deal with other people whom they can trust.
- People tend to judge other people and organizations on the basis of first impressions.

We must never forget that every time the client has any interaction with the clinic, they are reassessing the perceptions they have. The sum total of these assessments is a "new" overall impression of a practice. Perception is reality. For clients to readily accept our recommendations, they must believe that we are professionally competent. Because almost no client is capable of actually judging competence, that perception is grounded in areas in which they can make comparisons. Such things as friendliness, cleanliness, professionalism, state-of-the-art equipment, and time efficiency are common factors clients use in judging a veterinary practice.

We therefore gain clients' trust by making them feel important and confident they have made the right decisions for their pets. Treating the client as an individual, giving frequent compliments, respecting the client's opinion, using the client's name and pet's names often, being a good listener, respecting client's time, and expressing appreciation are all ways to make the client feel important.

Successful marketing depends on communicating with the client. Communication is incomplete without comprehension. We must talk in language that the client understands. Most clients will never tell a veterinarian if they don't understand something. The biggest barrier we have to overcome is assuming that a client understands what we are talking about. We must never assume a client knows what services the pet needs or what we can provide.

Children are great teachers of marketing ploys. All we really need to know to be successful in marketing our services we can learn from watching toddlers who want something.

- They are persistent.
- "No" always means "maybe."
- They are never embarrassed to ask.

Clients have three types of needs that a veterinarian must meet: professional, emotional, and consumer needs. The veterinarian satisfies these needs as follows:

1. Professional needs: Making the pet well and/or keeping it healthy.

2. Emotional needs: Making the client feel good about owning a pet, seeking veterinary attention, and choosing us to provide those services. This is the type of need that bonds most clients to return to the practice.

3. Consumer needs: These needs are most often the reasons a client first visits a practice. They include convenience, costs, and so on.

Successful marketing is an accumulation of many things. First and foremost is a perception by the client of our professional competence. Once the barrier has been broken, our marketing efforts must be directed toward "emotional selling." Our success depends on utilizing the following basic concepts to persuade the client of the need for the services we want to recommend:

- Show the benefits of the services to the pet.
- Show the benefits for accepting them now.
- Show the consequences for failing to accept them now.
- Show the benefits to the pet's owner.
- Show how the recommendation can benefit others.

Enthusiasm is essential for marketing services successfully. Enthusiasm comes from believing in what you recommend. The last four letters in *enthusiasm* stand for "I Am Sold Myself." The only thing more contagious than enthusiasm is apathy.

Enthusiasm is generated in the client through involvement. Some ways to involve the client are:

- Showing the problem on the pet's body.
- Explaining the importance of proper health care.
- Showing the client how to use the medication.
- Observing client efforts to use the medication.
- Scheduling frequent rechecks or telephone progress reports.

Smiling is one of the best ways to show enthusiasm. It breaks down barriers, drops defenses, increases credibility, shows we care, and defuses anger. The most important thing we can wear is a smile. We cannot afford to have a "bad day!"

We must understand that rejection is a part of successful marketing. The Coca-Cola Company sold only 400 bottles of their new beverage the first year. Marketing research indicates that it takes six to eight client interactions just to penetrate the subconscious. Sixteen to 18 interactions may be required to persuade the client to agree to our recommendations. The average consumer says "No" four times before saying "Yes."

Strategies for Marketing Ear Care and Otitis Treatment

Educate Yourself

As in all other facets of our veterinary education, we must first understand the abnormal condition and disease processes of the ear. The veterinarian should become adept at physical examination techniques and the appropriate laboratory evaluation of ear specimen smears and cultures. Surprisingly, a small amount of additional study time can greatly enhance one's professional abilities. Many references now contain in-depth chapters on ear conditions. This book, for example, can greatly enhance our visual perception of abnormalities that can be found in the ear. Almost all regional continuing education programs have full-day programs on ear diseases.

It is also important for the veterinarian to learn about the numerous products now available for both prevention and treatment of ear disease. The formulary contained in the Appendix of this book lists many products and their ingredients. The chapter on ototoxicity has a helpful guide to ingredients contained in products that may potentially cause problems if used in an animal with a ruptured eardrum. It is very important to understand not only what products are available but also their uses and contraindications.

Educate the Staff

Clients often talk to staff more than to the veterinarian. The veterinary staff is in the best position to "plant the seed," the idea of potential ear problems. The best salesman is the one already sold on the service. It is important that all staff members be educated as to the importance of proper ear care. Staff must understand the consequences of failures to catch ear disease early to completely resolve the ear problem before treatment is discontinued.

Staff must also understand the importance of *not* making a telephone or examination table diagnosis until the appropriate testing is performed by the veterinarian to determine the real problem. It is very hard for anyone to overcome wrong information provided to a client. Use of a video otoscope, such as the Video Vetscope (MedRx, Inc, Seminole, FL) in a practice allows all staff to see what the veterinarian sees deep in the ear canal on a video display. Staff can then "sell" clients on the idea of a more comprehensive ear examination when a client presents a pet for an ear problem or calls the practice to ask questions about a pet with an ear infection.

It is impossible for people to successfully market something they do not understand. The veterinarian should use all available commercial materials available to educate the staff. Many wall charts, pamphlets, books, and even ear models are available from suppliers of ear care products. Using a visual aid helps to learn about something not readily visualized on the animal.

Equip Yourself

Much of the instrumentation for ear care diagnostics and treatment is already in place. Client perception of professional competence is affected by the equipment used in the examination. Otoscopes should be in *every* examination room ready for use. Battery-operated otoscopes provide mobility in the clinic, and wall transformers avoid the embarrassment of dead batteries. Particular attention should be paid to having clean otoscope specula ready for immediate use. A new, innovative speculum cleaning device is available that contains a brush within a stainless steel cylinder filled with disinfectant. Having a speculum cleaner next to each otoscope provides a method of keeping the specula in each examination room clean and disinfected.

The expense of new equipment is relatively unimportant compared with the immediate cash flow that can result in most cases. Gross revenue enhancement is much more effective in increasing profits rather than trying to decrease expenses. Most practices find that once some new equipment is purchased, the caseload for use of that equipment increases immediately, if for no other reason than to "pay for it." The end-result is better client service and stimulation for the inquiring mind of the conscientious veterinarian.

A video otoscope is an excellent client education tool as well as an endoscopic instrument to facilitate ear procedures and treatment. Adequately visualizing a clear view of the inside of canine and feline ear canals and tympani is very difficult owing to the limits of the currently available otoscopes. Showing clients, staff, students, and other practitioners ear disease through a standard otoscope is an awkward demonstration.

A video otoscope employs new technology to expose the hidden world of ear examinations. Because the instrument is attached to a miniature video camera and video display, otic examinations can be visualized in real time on a video monitor for all to see. A color video printer allows "before and after" pictures of ear or dental treatments to be shown to the client at the time of diagnostics or when the pet is dismissed from the hospital after treatment. The photographs generated can provide information concerning pathologic conditions to clients so that they can make informed decisions about their pet's health care with the veterinarian's guidance.

Failing to look is much more of a problem in increasing potential income than a lack of knowledge. Using a video otoscope to examine the ears of every anesthetized pet (in the clinic for service unrelated to ear disease) greatly increases the discovery of additional medical problems present in an ear that would otherwise be overlooked. Problems found can then be photographed or videotaped for later view by the client. If the client can be contacted when the problem is discovered and he or she consents to the treatment, the photograph is factual evidence documenting the veterinarian's findings. If the client does not consent to treatment of an ear condition right away, the photograph serves as a constant reminder that the service needs to be scheduled. For difficult or extensive ear procedures, "before and after" pictures can enhance the client's perception of the value of the services performed.

The state-of-the-art video otoscope can also be used to add these images to the pet's computerized medical record and to generate future reminders to be mailed to the client. Adapters for the miniature video camera also allow other instruments in the hospital to be used to generate video pictures. A microscope adapter allows microscopic images to be video displayed on the monitor. An endoscope adapter allows the eyepiece of a flexible or rigid endoscope to attach to the miniature video camera, providing a real-time video image of the endoscopic examination.

Look for Problems

The foundation of a successful wellness program is a thorough history and physical examination of the patient. Time is required to be thorough. It is important to optimize time available for the veterinarian to make thorough examinations through staff delegation. Standardized medical history forms better ensure that a thorough history is obtained. Use of a pet examination "report card" further encourages a complete physical examination. Standard diagnostic protocols should be developed for dealing with ear abnormalities. With standardized protocols, staff can have the appropriate supplies and materials in the examination room ready for the veterinarian.

Ear cytological evaluation should become a routine procedure for all cases of otitis. Many cases of otitis are painful, and therefore sedation or anesthesia should be considered to ensure a thorough examination. Ear cleaning using anesthesia and a video otoscope allows for complete examination along the vertical and horizontal canals to look for disease. The eardrum and middle ear should be assessed in every patient. The veterinarian should never overlook a problem through failing to perform a thorough examination.

Educate the Client

People do not buy what they do not understand. Lacking knowledge about various treatment options, a client relies on price to make a choice. Because much ear disease lies deep in the ear, the pet owner may not even perceive that a problem exists. The old adage "show and tell to sell" is still true. Every client is an individual, and different. Everyone has a different "hot button," i.e., the particular stimulus triggering the client to accept a recommendation. This may be visual, auditory, tactile, olfactory, etc. Clients learn in different ways. It is important to find the hot button for each client. It is important to use education tools to ensure that the client understands the problem and what should be done about it.

Never assume that the client knows about all the services the pet needs and the veterinarian can provide. The veterinarian should make sure to use all the senses to enhance the client's perception of an abnormality:

1. Show the problem through the otoscope, teaching head otoscope, or the video otoscope. Reddened, inflamed ears are easy to see.
2. Have the client smell the odor.
3. Have the client feel the swollen or bony ear canals.
4. If the pet whines when the ears are manipulated or examined with the otoscope, explain that ear infections are painful; compare them to human ear infections.

Other visual aids are available:

- Diagrams of the ear's anatomy framed and placed on the wall in each examination room.
- Wall poster of photographs of dog and cat ear diseases.

- Looseleaf notebooks in each examination room with details of ear diseases and surgical procedures.
- Brochures from product suppliers.
- "Silent" reception room tools, such as video monitors with films of ear diseases
- Ear models
- Handouts on clinic letterhead with a diagram of the ear, to be used to show where in the ear the problem lies. The veterinarian should make it standard policy that no client ever leaves the clinic without a handout about something; handouts become miniature billboards reminding the client of the veterinarian's recommendations.

The most important educational tool is staff and veterinarian interaction with clients. Staff should be trained in the proper use of pictures and models to explain ear disease. Much of the client education effort can be delegated to staff.

Everyone must understand the serious potential problems that otitis can cause. To increase client compliance, relate otitis to the following ideas:

1. Otitis hurts: It can be very painful. Many pets with painful ear infections may show behavioral changes, such as aggression, from the pain. Compare pain to that of human ear infections.

2. Otitis stinks: A stinky pet may well not stay in the house for long. Pets relegated to the backyard most often do not get the best care from that time on.

3. Otitis is infection: Any infection can be a "seed" for infection elsewhere in the body. Infection can rupture the eardrum and allow the spread of disease to the middle ear, inner ear, or even the brain stem.

4. Otitis can cause a loss of hearing: Hearing loss may occur from either swollen, stenotic ear canals, otitis media, or inner ear infection.

5. Otitis can cause neurological signs: Head tilt, rapid eye movements (nystagmus), and circling may indicate that the infection has moved into nervous tissues.

6. Otitis can result in future expense: Many chronic, recurrent ear infections are actually the same infection that has never been properly treated and followed up until the ear is back to normal.

Consider the possibility of a heightened anxiety level in the client during the office visit. Minimizing this anxiety allows the client to concentrate more on what you are saying. In many cases, it is best to have the pet held in another area of the hospital while consulting with pet owners.

Methods of entertaining children should also be available in veterinary clinics to minimize client distraction. Successful client education requires an environment conducive to learning. Anxiety can also develop from a client's perception that the examination "hurts" the pet. The veterinarian should not hesitate to recommend sedation or anesthesia so that a thorough examination may be performed.

It is also important to educate the client about the many products available that have the potential for enhancing the ear's resistance to infection (ear cleaners, for example). Educate the client—and then let him or her decide. Every client decision should be an educated decision.

Most treatment failures are a result of poor client compliance with treatment at home. Successful outcomes require that the clients understand the importance of proper home treatment. Written home care instructions should always be provided as well as discussed with the client. Proper administration of the medication should be demonstrated, and the client should then be asked to demonstrate proficiency with the procedures. Many patients with symptomatic otitis are resistant to manipulation of their ears. If the client cannot medicate the pet at home, the veterinarian should offer to provide the treatment in the clinic twice daily as a drop-in procedure. After a few days of proper treatment, the pet will feel more comfortable and the pain is reduced, so the owner can take over treatment at home. The veterinarian and staff should be sure to praise client efforts; everyone likes compliments. Compliance with home care should always be discussed during telephone progress checks.

Make Your Services Convenient

Convenience rules the world today. The astute veterinarian offers such services as pet drop-off and late pick-up. Treatment procedures, such as topical medications should be started during the initial visit to better ensure client compliance. All needed services should be scheduled for a time most convenient for the client; in most cases, that is the initial time of presentation. The veterinarian demonstrates respect for the client's time and that of clients with late appointments by recommending that a pet be left in the clinic for a few hours while complete diagnostic evaluations and therapeutic procedures are performed. The client will appreciate the explanation that it would be more convenient to perform all needed services because the pet is already there. Staff should be trained to schedule a specific dismissal appointment time to minimize client waiting time at the time of dismissal. An extended wait to check out can increase client frustration and level of anxiety.

Price for Your Market

The major cause of relapsing otitis is the failure to recheck. A line item on a client's bill called "otitis recheck package" could be developed to include the recheck fee, sedation, ear swab and evaluations, and treatment. Discounting merely hints to a client that the veterinarian's services are overpriced. These services, if put into a package, should not be discounted. Rather, the package should be given a separate service code in the computer with the total fee charged for these procedures at the discounted rate lumped into one fee. Even though the effect is the same, the client perceives total fee to be reasonable and there is no hint of discounting.

In matters of pricing, there are two kinds of fools: those who charge too much and those who charge too little. Fortunately, veterinary ear services are not comparison-shopped for price. Therefore, it is a simple matter for the veterinarian to price the procedures to fit the particular practice and clientele. Pricing is no longer based on what it costs to provide a service, but rather what the client perceives is "fair." Services that pet owners shop for by telephone, such as spays, neuters, and vaccines, must be priced competitively to prevent the perception that the veterinarian's other services are overpriced.

Ear therapeutics is one area of practice in which the higher total fees charged make up for some of the lower-priced services that must be provided for a practice to remain competitively priced. On the client invoice, the fee for each component of the service provided (external ear canal flush and suction, middle ear flush and suction, foreign body removal, biopsy, etc.) should be shown, in addition to the fees for examination, cytological evaluation, sedation, culture, and medications. The fee charged for each procedure is perceived by the client to indicate the difficulty of performing that procedure. Treatment of ear disease often requires a number of different procedures to be performed on the same patient.

The veterinarian's fees should always be related to value. Clients should always leave with tangible evidence of the intangible services; examples for ear disease are a pet examination report card or a picture of the ear canal taken with the video otoscope. These suggestions enhance the perceived value of the services rendered to the client. Clients must perceive that the veterinarian's services are worth the fees charged.

Remind Clients

As already stated, six to eight client interactions are required just to penetrate the subconscious. The strategy of "planting the seed" must be understood by everyone in the practice.

Most people are uncomfortable making quick decisions. Even a pet's chronic renal failure may be an acute diagnosis for the owner, although the doctor knows that it has been present for months to years. The veterinarian should:

- Go slowly, giving the client time to weigh the potential disadvantages of *not* accepting the recommendations.
- Give the client a reason to act promptly (pain relief and patient comfort).

- Show the client how he or she as well as the pet will benefit (reduction in offensive odor).

Today's veterinary client has the absolute right to be demanding. It is important that all staff members understand that the clients must always be given the opportunity to provide the best level of health care available for their beloved family member. Veterinarians must *never* be the reason that any pet does not have the opportunity for the best ear care the profession has to offer.

Computer searches of the client base can produce lists of patients with past otitis problems for targeted marketing efforts. Even offering complimentary rechecks for these cases will result in significant findings for which additional services and products are needed. The key is simply getting the pets presented for examination so the doctor can find the problems and then market the needed services.

Follow-Up

It is surprising how many veterinarians are willing to allow a client to spend large sums of money on ear diagnostics and therapy and then rely on the client's impression to determine the pet's response to treatment. A phone call to a client to check on the pet's progress in 24 to 48 hours impresses the client. It reflects a caring attitude and stresses the importance the doctor has placed on resolving the pet's ear disease.

Clients respond much better when they are treated nicely from the start and are made to feel that they are an important part of their pet's future well-being. Scheduling and charging for follow-up examinations and diagnostic testing greatly enhances the client bonding rate to the practice, builds client trust, and ensures administration of appropriate therapy. Staff should *always* schedule the recheck appointment and ensure that reminders are entered into the computer before the client leaves. The veterinarian should also consider sending reminder notes to clients about procedures they did not accept at the time of the initial recommendation. For a dog diagnosed with heartworms, for example, a future reminder would be sent for heartworm treatment. For a dog with severe wax accumulation in the ear canals, a reminder should be for an ear flush or waxball extraction at a future date. All pets receiving long-term medication require periodic rechecks.

Become Creative

The veterinarian who wishes to improve or enlarge a practice should consider the following activities:

- Plan a staff meeting to discuss ear care, and ask the staff for ideas.
- Write an article for a local newspaper on pet ear care.

- Position the practice as an ear care clinic.
- Place messages on your outside marquee reader board to generate questions if this type of outside sign is being used.
- Develop relationships with local groomers to increase the number of referrals for ear disease.

It is now known that a major reason clients do not request more dental services is a fear of anesthesia for their pets. Clients remember the pet that was lost 20 years ago during a "routine" spaying. They do not understand the advances made in veterinary anesthetics, sedatives, and analgesics. The veterinarian and staff should be careful not to create undue anxiety in clients by overemphasizing the "risks" of anesthesia needed for proper ear cleaning. Clients must always be informed of the inherent risks possible with all drugs used, but they must also understand the need for these drugs in painful ear conditions. Client perception is greatly altered by simply using the term "sedation" instead of "anesthesia." Using reversible sedatives or analgesics when possible also lessens client anxiety. However, the use of anesthetics may be needed, however, and the veterinarian must lessen the client's anxiety with proper communication. A written consent should always be obtained when sedation or anesthesia is a requirement for proper ear treatment.

Conclusion

Marketing ear care is one of the most professional services veterinarians can offer. Clients perceive the veterinarian as an expert. More ear disease is missed because veterinarians do not take the time to look. It is not that veterinarians do not know that ear disease is present; they are not specifically looking for it. Ear care is one of the services with an extremely high potential to enlarge a practice. Current estimates indicate that 15% to 20% of all canine patients and 4% to 6% of all feline patients presented to the veterinarian have ear disease. A little quick arithmetic reveals that the income potential for marketing ear services is enormous (see box).

MAKING EAR CARE A PROFIT CENTER IN THE VETERINARY CLINIC)

To show how profitable developing a high-quality ear care program can be, consider the typical clinic client base of 2500 canine patients and 1000 feline patients.

Applying estimates of ear disease rates in an existing patient base (left) show the following potential for ear disease treatment (right):

10%–20% of canine patients have ear disease	250 to 500 patients
4%–6% of feline patients have ear disease	40 to 60 patients

Between 290 and 560 patients in the practice have current ear disease.

Minimum services needed and suggested fees to perform a thorough ear examination:

Office visit and physical examination	$28
Ear swab cytological evaluation	$20
Sedation/reversal	$30
External ear flush and suction on each ear	$30
Total	$108

The income potential from *examination only* can generate from **$31,320** (290 patients × $108) to **$54,648** (560 patients × $108).

Add fees for any treatments, drugs, additional tests, surgical procedures, follow-up, and so on, and the income stream continues to increase.

There is probably sufficient ear disease present in the patient bases of most practices to keep a veterinarian busy full time. The real question is whether the practitioner is willing to dedicate himself or herself to finding all the ear problems and then educating the clients about them. Upon the veterinarian's recommendation, most pet owners do decide to have the recommended service performed. That is all there is to successfully marketing high-quality ear care in a veterinary practice.

It is the veterinarian's professional, ethical, and moral duty to recommend everything the pet needs. It is good medicine, and it is good business.

Appendix
Ear Product Formulary

This formulary is presented as a guide to products available for treating ear disease. The products listed are for *topical use* in the ear canal unless indicated otherwise. Many topical formulations are compounded mixtures containing ingredients that may be potentially ototoxic when there is no eardrum. Consult the manufacturer for the recommendation for use when the eardrum is perforated.

The organization of the formulary is by function or mode of action. Ingredients are categorized as anti-inflammatory, antibacterial, anti-fungal, miticidal, ear cleaners, and drying agents. Some formulations have more than one function and may be listed again in the appropriate sections. Under each category, the generic ingredient, the trade name, and the manufacturers are listed. The proprietary names and active ingredients of products are listed after the ingredients.

Active Ingredients of Ear Products, Listed by Function

Potent Anti-Inflammatory Agents

Betamethasone 0.1%	Genta-Otic	Vetus
	Gentaved Otic	Vedco
	Gentocin Otic	Schering
	Otomax	Schering
	Topagen	Schering
	Tri-Otic	Med-Pharmex
Betamethasone 0.64 mg	Lotrisone	Schering
Dexamethasone 0.1%	Decadron Phosphate	Merck
	Tobradex	Alcon
	Tresaderm	Merial
Fluocinolone 0.01%	Synotic Otic	Ft. Dodge

Moderate Anti-Inflammatory Agents

Isoflupredone acetate 0.1%	Neo-Predef	Pharmacia & Upjohn
	Tritop	Pharmacia & Upjohn
Triamcinolone acetonide 0.1%	Animax	Pharmaderm
	Coly-Mycin S Otic	Parke-Davis
	Cortisporin Otic	Glaxo Wellcome
	Derma 4 Ointment	Pfizer
	Dermalone	Vedco
	Derma-Vet	Med-Pharmex
	Forte Topical	Upjohn & Pharmacia
	Neo-Predef	Upjohn & Pharmacia
	Panolog	Solvay

Mild Anti-Inflammatory Agents

Hydrocortisone acetate 0.2%	Forte Topical	Pharmacia & Upjohn
Hydrocortisone 1%	Bur-O-Cort	Q.A. Labs
	Burotic HC	Allerderm
	Cipro HC Otic	Bayer Pharmaceutical
	Clear X Ear Drying Solution	DVM
	Coly-Mycin S Otic	Parke-Davis
	CORT/ASTRIN	Vedco
	Cortisporin Otic	Glaxo Wellcome
	Epiotic HC	Allerderm
	VōSol HC Otic	Wallace
Prednisolone 0.17%	Chlora-Otic	Vetus
	Liquichlor	Evsco

Antibacterials

Acetic acid– boric acid	DermaPet Ear/ Skin Cleanser	DermaPet, Inc.
Chloramphenicol	Clora-Otic	Vetus
	Chloromycetin Otic	Parke-Davis
	Liquichlor	Evsco
Ciprofloxacin	Cipro HC Otic	Bayer Pharmaceuticals
Colistin	Coly-Mycin S Otic	Parke-Davis
Enrofloxacin	Baytril injection	Bayer

(Mix 2 mL in 13 mL artificial tears or saline)

Gentamicin	Genta-Otic	Vetus
	Gentaved Otic	Vedco
	Gentocin Otic	Schering
	Otomax	Schering
	Topagen Ointment	Schering
	Tri-Otic	Med-Pharmex
Neomycin	Animax	Pharmaderm
	Coly-Mycin S Otic	Parke-Davis
	Cortisporin Otic	Glaxo Wellcome
	Derma 4 Ointment	Pfizer
	Dermalone	Vedco
	Derma-Vet	Med-Pharmex
	Forte Topical	Upjohn & Pharmacia

Neomycin *(continued)*	Neo-Predef	Upjohn & Pharmacia
	Panolog	Solvay
	Quadritop	Vetus
	Tresaderm	Merial
	Tritop	Upjohn & Pharmacia
Ofloxacin	Floxin Otic	Daiichi
Polymyxin B Sulfate	Cortisporin	Glaxo-Wellcome
	Forte Topical	Upjohn & Pharmacia
	Otobiotic Otic	Schering-Plough
Silver sulfadiazine 0.1%	Silvadene Creme	Marion

(Mix 1.5 mL cream in 13.5 mL distilled water)

Ticarcillin	Ticar 1 g vial	SmithKline Beecham

(Mix with 2 mL sterile water. Add 0.5 mL of this solution to 15 mL artificial tears or saline. Keep refrigerated. Use as ear drop for 1 week, then discard remaining solution.)
Freeze the remainder in 0.5-mL increments for future use; good for 90 days frozen.)

Tobramycin	Tobradex Ophthalmic	Alcon
TrisEDTA	TrizEDTA	DermaPet, Inc.

Antifungals

Acetic acid–boric acid	DermaPet Ear/ Skin Cleanser	DermaPet, Inc.
Clotrimazole 1%	Lotrimin AF	Schering-Plough
	Lotrisone	Schering-Plough
	Otomax	Schering
	Tri-Otic	Med-Pharmex
Miconazole 1%	Conofite	Mallinckrodt
	Micazole	Vetus
	Miconosol	Med-Pharmex
Nystatin 100,000 U/mL	Animax	Pharmaderm
	Derma-4	Pfizer
	Dermalone	Vedco
	Derma-Vet	Med-Pharmex
	Panolog	Solvay
	Quadritop	Vetus

| *Zinc undecylenate* | Fungi-dry-ear | Q.A. Labs |

Miticidals

| *Fipronil* | Frontline Top Spot | Merial |
| *Ivermectin 1% injectable* | Ivomec 1% | Merial |

      (0.1 mL/10 lb subcutaneously every 2 weeks for 3 injections)

Pyrethrins	Aurimite	Schering
	Cerumite	Evsco
	Eradimite	Solvay
	Mita-Clear	Pfizer
	Nolvamite with Nolvasan	Ft. Dodge
	Oticare-M Ear Mite Treatment	ARC
	Otomite Plus	Allerderm
Rotenone 0.12%	Mitaplex-R	Tomlyn
Rotenone 0.12% & cube resins 0.16%	Ear Mite Lotion	DurVet
	Ear Miticide	Vedco
	Ear Miticide	Phoenix
Thiabendazole	Tresaderm	Merial

Ear Products Listed by Trade Names

Animax Ointment
Active ingredients: Combines nystatin, neomycin sulfate, thiostrepton, and triamcinolone acetonide in a nonirritating polyethylene and mineral oil base.

Aurimite
Active ingredients: Dioctyl sodium sulfosuccinate 1.952% w/w, benzocaine 1.952% w/w, technical piperonyl butoxide 0.49% w/w, pyrethrins 0.04% w/w, inert ingredients 95.566%.

Baytril Injection Solution
Each mL of injection solution contains enrofloxacin 22.7 mg, *n*-butyl alcohol 30 mg, potassium hydroxide for pH adjustment, and water for injection, q.s.

Bur-O-Cort 2:1
Active ingredients: Each mL contains Burow's solution (astringent) 20 mg, hydrocortisone (anti-inflammatory, antipruritic) 10 mg.

Burotic HC
Active ingredients: Hydrocortisone, 1%. Other ingredients: propylene glycol, water, Burow's solution, acetic acid, benzalkonium chloride.

CERUMITE
Active ingredients: Squalane (hexamethyltetracosane) 25.00%, pyrethrins 0.05%, technical piperonyl butoxide 0.50%, inert ingredients 74.45%.

Chlora-Otic
Active ingredients: Each mL contains chloramphenicol 4.2 mg, prednisolone 1.7 mg, tetracaine 4.2 mg, squalane 0.21 mL.

Chloromycetin Otic
Active ingredients: Each mL contains 5 mg (0.5%) chloramphenicol in propylene glycol.

Cipro HC Otic
Active ingredients: Each mL contains ciprofloxacin HCl (equivalent to 2 mg ciprofloxacin), 10 mg hydrocortisone, and 9 mg benzyl alcohol as a preservative.

Clear X Ear Drying Solution
Active ingredients: Acetic acid 2.5%, colloidal sulfur 2%, hydrocortisone 1%.

Coly-Mycin S Otic
Active ingredients: Each mL contains colistin base activity, 3 mg (as the sulfate), neomycin base activity, 3.3 mg (as the sulfate), hydrocortisone acetate 10 mg (1%), thonzonium bromide, 0.5 mg (0.5%), with polysorbate 80, acetic acid, sodium acetate buffered at pH 5.

Conofite Lotion
Active ingredients: 1.15% miconazole nitrate (equivalent to 1% miconazole base by weight), polyethylene glycol 400, and ethyl alcohol 55%.

CORT/ASTRIN Solution
Active ingredients: Each mL contains Burow's solution 20 mg, hydrocortisone 10 mg in a water-miscible propylene glycol base.

Cortisporin Otic Solution
Active ingredients: Each mL contains polymyxin B sulfate 10,000 units, neomycin sulfate 3.5 mg neomycin base, and hydrocortisone 10 mg (0.1%). The vehicle contains potassium metabisulfate 0.1% and the inactive ingredients cupric sulfate, glycerin, hydrochloric acid, propylene glycol, and water for injection.

Decadron Phosphate 0.1%
Active ingredients: Each mL contains 1 mg dexamethasone phosphate. Inactive ingredients: creatinine, sodium citrate, sodium borate, polysor-

bate 80, disodium edetate, hydrochloric acid to adjust pH, and water for injection.

Derma 4 Ointment
Composition: Each mL contains 100,000 units of nystatin, neomycin sulfate (equivalent to 2.5 mg of neomycin base), 2500 units of thiostrepton, and 1.0 mg of triamcinolone acetonide. Inert ingredients include Plastibase 50-weight,* 20%; and mineral oil USP, 80%.

Dermalone Ointment
Active ingredients: Each mL contains nystatin 100,000 units, neomycin sulfate (equivalent to neomycin base) 2.5 mg, thiostrepton 2500 units, triamcinolone acetonide 1.0 mg, polyethylene and mineral oil gel base.

Derma-Vet Ointment
Active ingredients: Each mL contains nystatin 100,000 units, neomycin sulfate (equivalent to neomycin base) 2.5 mg, thiostrepton 2500 units, triamcinolone acetonide 1.0 mg.

Epi-otic HC
Active ingredients: Contains hydrocortisone 1%, lactic acid, and PCMX in a surface acting vehicle.

Ear Mite Lotion
Active ingredients: Rotenone 0.12%, cube resins 0.16%, inert ingredients 99.72%.

Ear Miticide (Vedco)
Active ingredients: Rotenone 0.12%, cube resins 0.16%, inert ingredients 99.72%.

Ear Miticide (Phoenix)
Active ingredients: Rotenone 0.12%, cube resins 0.16%, inert ingredients 99.72%.

Eradimite
Active ingredients: Pyrethrins 0.15%, piperonyl butoxide, technical, 1.50%, inert ingredients 98.35%.

Floxin Otic
Active ingredients: 0.3% (3 mg/mL) ofloxacin with benzalkonium chloride 0.0025%, sodium chloride 0.9%, and water for injection. Hydrochloric acid and sodium hydroxide are added to adjust the pH to 6.5.

Forte-Topical
Active ingredients: Contains (per mL) 2 mg hydrocortisone acetate, 1.25 mg hydrocortisone sodium succinate, 25 mg neomycin sulfate (equivalent

*Plastibase Trademark of E.R. Squibb & Sons, Princeton, N.J.

to 17.5 mg of neomycin), 10,000 IU penicillin G procaine, 5000 units polymyxin B sulfate, and 5 mg chlorobutanol anhydrous (chloral derivative), in a special bland vehicle.

Frontline Top Spot
Active ingredients: Fipronil: 5-amino-1-(2,6-dichloro-4-(trifluoromethyl) phenyl)-4-((1,R,S)-(trifluoromethyl)sulfinyl)-1-H-pyrazole-3-carbonitrile 9.7%. Inert ingredients 90.3%.

Fungi-dry-ear
Active ingredients: Isopropyl alcohol, de-ionized water, silicon dioxide, zinc undecylenate (undecylenic acid), methyl salicylate, PEG 75 lanolin oil, sucrose octyl acetate, polysorbate 60, propylene glycol, acetic acid, FD & C blue #1.

Genta-Otic Solution
Active ingredients: Each mL contains gentamicin sulfate equivalent to 3 mg gentamicin base, betamethasone valerate equivalent to 1 mg betamethasone, 1.0 mg hydroxyethylcellulose, 2.5 mg glacial acetic acid, 200 mg purified water, 19% ethanol, 9.4 mg benzyl alcohol as preservative, 300 mg glycerin and propylene glycol q.s.

Gentaved Otic Solution
Active ingredients: Each mL contains gentamicin sulfate equivalent to 3 mg gentamicin base, betamethasone valerate equivalent to 1 mg betamethasone, 1.0 mg hydroxyethylcellulose, 2.5 mg glacial acetic acid, 200 mg purified water, 19% ethanol, 9.4 mg benzyl alcohol as preservative, 300 mg glycerin, and propylene glycol q.s.

Gentocin Otic Solution
Active ingredients: Each mL contains gentamicin sulfate equivalent to 3 mg gentamicin base, betamethasone valerate equivalent to 1 mg betamethasone, 1.0 mg hydroxyethylcellulose, 2.5 mg glacial acetic acid, 200 mg purified water, 19% ethanol, 9.4 mg benzyl alcohol as preservative, 300 mg glycerin, and propylene glycol q.s.

Ivomec 1% Injection for Cattle and Swine
Active ingredients: Contains 1% ivermectin, 40% glycerol formal, and propylene glycol, q.s. at 100%.

Liquichlor
Active ingredients: Each mL contains chloramphenicol 4.2 mg, prednisolone 1.7 mg, tetracaine 4.2 mg, squalane 0.21 mL.

Lotrisone
Active ingredients: Each gram contains 10.0 mg clotrimazole, 0.64 mg betamethasone diproprionate (equivalent to 0.5 mg betamethasone) in a hydrophilic emollient creme consisting of purified water, mineral oil, white petrolatum, cetostearyl alcohol, cetareth-30, propylene glycol, sodium phosphate, monobasic, and phosphoric acid.

Micazole Lotion 1%
Active ingredients: Contains 1.15% miconazole nitrate (equivalent to 1% miconazole base by weight), polyethylene glycol 400, and ethyl alcohol 55%.

Miconosol Lotion 1%
Active ingredients: Contains 1.15% miconazole nitrate (equivalent to 1% miconazole base by weight), polyethylene glycol 400, and ethyl alcohol 55%.

Mita-Clear
Active ingredients: Pyrethrins 0.15%, piperonyl butoxide, technical, 1.50%, N-octyl bicycloheptene dicarboximide 0.50%, di-n-propyl isocinchomeronate 1.00%. Inert ingredients: 96.85%.

MITAPLEX-R
Active ingredients: Rotenone 0.120%. Inert ingredients: 99.880%.

Neo-Predef
Active ingredients: Each gram contains isoflupredone acetate 1 mg (0.1%), and the antibiotic neomycin sulfate, 5 mg (0.5%) (equivalent to 3.5 mg neomycin); also anhydrous lanolin, white petrolatum, and mineral oil. Chlorobutanol (chloral derivative) 0.65% added as preservative.

Nolvamite
Active ingredients: Pyrethrin 0.10%, piperonyl butoxide, technical, 1.05%, inert ingredients 98.85%. Contains Nolvasan as a preservative.

Oticare-M Ear Mite Treatment
Active ingredients: Pyrethrins 0.15%, piperonyl butoxide technical 1.50%. Inert ingredients: 98.35%.

Otomax
Active ingredients: Each gram contains gentamicin sulfate veterinary equivalent to 3 mg gentamicin base; betamethasone valerate, USP equivalent to 1 mg betamethasone; and 10 mg clotrimazole, USP in a mineral oil–based system containing a plasticized hydrocarbon gel.

Otomite Plus
Active ingredients: Pyrethrins 0.15%, technical piperonyl butoxide 1.50%, N-octyl bicycloheptene dicarboximide 0.5%, di-n-propyl isocincho-meronate 1.0%. Inert ingredients: 96.85%.

Panolog Ointment
Active ingredients: Contains nystatin, neomycin sulfate, thiostrepton, and triamcinolone acetonide in a nonirritating protective vehicle, Plastibase (plasticized hydrocarbon gel), a polyethylene and mineral oil gel base.

Quadritop Ointment
Ingredients: Each mL contains nystatin 100,000 units, neomycin sulfate (equivalent to neomycin base) 2.5 mg, thiostrepton 2500 units, triamcinolone acetonide 1.0 mg.

Silvadene Creme 1%
Active ingredients: Each gram contains 10 mg micronized silver sulfadiazine. The cream vehicle consists of white petrolatum, stearyl alcohol, isopropyl myristate, sorbitan monooleate, polyoxyl 40 stearate, propylene glycol and water.

Synotic Otic Solution
Active ingredients: Each mL of the solution contains 0.01% fluocinolone acetonide (6a,9a-difluoro-11b,16a,17,21-tetrahydroxypregna-1,4-diene-3, 20-dione, cyclic 16,17-acetal with acetone) and 60% dimethyl sulfoxide in propylene glycol and citric acid.

Ticar sterile powder for intramuscular or intravenous injection
Active ingredients: Ticarcillin is a semisynthetic injectible penicillin derivative supplied as a white to pale yellow powder for reconstitution.

Tobradex Suspension
Each mL contains: Active ingredients: tobramycin 0.3% (3 mg) and dexamethasone 0.1% (1 mg). Preservative: benzalkonium chloride 0.01%. Inactive ingredients: tyloxapol, edetate disodium, sodium chloride, hydroxyethyl cellulose, sodium sulfate, sulfuric acid and/or sodium hydroxide (to adjust pH) and purified water.

Topagen Ointment
Active ingredients: Each gram contains gentamicin sulfate veterinary equivalent to 3 mg gentamicin base, betamethasone valerate equivalent to 1 mg betamethasone, and sesame oil in a special gel base composed of polyethylene and mineral oil; benzyl alcohol is the preservative.

Tresaderm
Active ingredients: Each mL contains thiabendazole 40 mg, dexamethasone 1 mg, neomycin (from neomycin sulfate) 3.2 mg. Inactive ingredients: Glycerin propylene glycol, purified water, hypophosphorous acid, calcium hypophosphite, about 8.5% ethyl alcohol, and about 0.5% benzyl alcohol.

Tri-Otic
Active ingredients: Each gram of gentamicin-betamethasone-clotrimazole ointment contains gentamicin sulfate USP equivalent to 3 mg gentamicin base; betamethasone valerate USP equivalent to 1 mg betamethasone; and 10 mg clotrimazole USP in a mineral oil–based system containing a plasticized hydrocarbon gel.

Tritop
Active ingredients: Contains in each gram the potent anti-inflammatory agent isoflupredone acetate 1 mg (0.1%), the antibiotic neomycin sulfate,

5 mg (0.5%) (equivalent to 3.5 mg neomycin), and the topical anesthetic tetracaine hydrochloride, 5 mg (0.5%).

Vōsol HC Otic
Active ingredients: Solution of acetic acid 2% in a propylene glycol vehicle containing propylene glycol acetate (3%) and hydrocortisone (1%).

Ear Cleaners, Listed by Trade Name

Ace-otic (Vetus)
Active ingredients: Acetic acid 2.0%, lactic acid 2.7%, salicylic acid 0.1%. In a pH-buffered at 2.3 surface-active vehicle containing docusate sodium (DSS) and propylene glycol.

Adams pan-otic (Pfizer)
Active ingredients: Purified water USP, isopropyl alcohol, aloe vera, diazolidinyl urea, methylparaben, propylparaben, dioctyl sodium sulfosuccinate, octoxynol, sodium lauryl sulfate, parachlorometaxylenol, propylene glycol USP, fragrance, tetrasodium EDTA, FD&C blue #1.

Aloacetic Ear Rinse (DVM)
Ingredients: Water, acetic acid, nonoxynol-12, fragrance, methylparaben, DMDM hydantoin, aloe vera gel, FD&C yellow #5, FD&C blue #1.

Burotic (Allerderm)
Active ingredients: Contains propylene glycol, water, Burow's solution, acetic acid, benzalkonium chloride.

Cerulytic (Allerderm)
Active ingredients: Contains benzyl alcohol and butylated hydroxytoluene in a propylene glycoldicaprylate/dicaprate base with fragrance.

Cerumene (Evsco)
Active ingredients: Contains cerumene (squalane) 25% in an isopropyl myristate liquid petrolatum base.

Clear X Ear Cleansing Solution (DVM)
Active ingredients: Contains dioctyl sodium sulfosuccinate 6.5%, urea peroxide 6%.

Corium 20 (VRx)
Active ingredients: Contains purified water USP, SDA-40B 23%, glycerol triesterified with fatty acids, glycerine USP, fragrance and B.H.A.

Corium TX (VRx)
Active ingredients: Pramoxine HCl (1%). Also contains purified water USP, SDA-40B 23%, glycerol tri-esterified with fatty acids, glycerine USP, Tween 80, fragrance, B.H.A.

DermaPet Ear/Skin Cleanser (DermaPet, Inc.)
Active ingredients: A multicleanse, acetic and boric acid solution with surfactants.

EarMed Cleansing Solution & Wash (Davis)
Active ingredients: 50A 40B alcohol, propylene glycol, cocamidopropyl phosphatidyl and PE dimonium chloride.

EarOxide Ear Cleaner (Tomlyn)
Active ingredients: Contains carbamide peroxide 6.5% in a stabilized glycerin base.

Epiotic Ear Cleanser (Allerderm)
Ingredients: Lactic acid and salicylic acid are present in encapsulated (Spherulites) and free forms. Chitosanide is present in encapsulated form. PCMX, propylene glycol, and sodium docusate are present in free form. Also contains water, fragrance, and FD&C blue #1.

Fresh-Ear (Q.A. Labs)
Active ingredients: Contains deionized water, isopropyl alcohol, propylene glycol, glycerine, fragrance, salicylic acid, PEG 75 lanolin oil, lidocaine hydrochloride, boric acid, acetic acid, FD&C blue #1.

Gent-L-Clens (Schering)
Active ingredients: Contains lactic acid and salicylic acid in a propylene glycol surface-acting vehicle preserved with PCMX.

Nolvasan Otic (Ft. Dodge)
Active ingredients: Contains special solvent and surfactant.

Oticalm Cleansing Solution (DVM)
Active ingredients: Contains benzoic acid, malic acid, salicylic acid, oil of eucalyptus in a soothing solubilizing vehicle.

Otic Clear (Butler)
Active ingredients: Contains deionized water, isopropyl alcohol, propylene glycol, glycerine, fragrance, salicylic acid, PEG 75 lanolin oil, lidocaine hydrochloride, boric acid, acetic acid, FD&C blue #1.

Oticlean A Ear Cleaning Solution (ARC)
Active ingredients: Contains 35% isopropyl alcohol, boric acid, salicylic acid, fragrance, PEG 75, lanolin oil, acetic acid, propylene glycol, glycerine, and FD&C blue #1.

Oticlens (Pfizer)
Active ingredients: A clear, colorless liquid with an approximate pH of 2.3 prepared from the following active ingredients: propylene glycol, malic acid, benzoic acid, and salicylic acid.

Otipan Cleansing Solution (Harlmen)
Active ingredients: Contains propylene glycol, hydroxypropyl cellulose, octoxynol, and a phosphate buffer system (phosphoric acid and potassium hydroxide). The pH is adjusted to 2.5 or less.

Otisol (Wysong)
Active ingredients: Contains copper chelate of chlorophyl, essential oils of eucalyptus, peppermint, cajeput, juniper, wintergreen, clove, jojoba oil, aloe vera extract, benzocaine, carbolic acid, and natural oleoresins, menthol in a coconut soap, sodium metasilicate, isopropranol base. Stabilized with rosemary extract and vitamin E.

Otisol O (Wysong)
Active ingredients: Contains copper chelate of chlorophyll, jojoba oil, aloe vera, arnica, and essential oils of eucalyptus, peppermint, cajeput, juniper, wintergreen, clove, and menthol in a base of extra virgin olive oil stabilized with Wysong oxherphol (tocopherol epimers of vitamin E, botanical oleoresins, ascorbate oxidase, and glutathione peroxidase).

Otocetic Solution (Vedco)
Active ingredients: Contains 2% acetic acid with surfactants.

Wax-O-Sol (Life Science)
Active ingredients: Contains 25% hexamethyltetracosane in mineral oil.

Ear Drying Products

CLEARX Ear Drying Solution (DVM)
Active ingredients: Contains acetic acid 2.5%, colloidal sulfur 2%, hydrocortisone 1%.

Oticare B Drying Creme (ARC)
Ingredients: Contains 70% isopropyl alcohol, silicon dioxide, salicylic acid, boric acid, fragrance, polysorbate 60, zinc oxide, talc, PEG 75 lanolin oil, sucrose octyl acetate, acetic acid, propylene glycol, FD&C blue #1.

Subject Index

Note: Page numbers in *italics* indicate figures. Page numbers followed by *t* indicate tables.

A

Acetazolamide, ototoxicity of, 147*t*
Acetic acid, ototoxicity of, 149*t,* 151
Acetic acid–boric acid, antibacterials
    containing, 241
  antifungals containing, 242
  solution of (DermaPet Ear/Skin Cleaner),
    bathing procedure using, 216
  for *Malassezia* otitis externa, 109–110
Acoustic meatus, external, 5, 13, *13–15*
  innervation of, 8
  stenosis of, 50, *50*
  internal, *19,* 20
Acoustic nerve. See *Cranial nerve VIII*
  (acoustic).
Actinomycin C, ototoxicity of, 147*t*
Actinomycin D, ototoxicity of, 147*t*
Adenocarcinoma, ceruminous gland, in
    cats, *71–72,* 75
  in dogs, 75, 195
  incidence of, 75
  sebaceous gland, in cats, 75
Adenoma(s), ceruminous gland, *49*
  ear canal occlusion by, 54, *54*
  gross examination of, 72, *73*
  in cats, 75, 195
  in dogs, 195
  incidence of, 75
  ulcerated, *70*
  sebaceous gland, in cats, 195
  in dogs, 75, 195
Adrenocortical hyperplasia, in dogs,
    185–186
Aeroallergy, 115–116
  clinical signs of, 116

Aeroallergy *(Continued)*
  diagnosis of, 116
  incidence of, 116
  otitis caused by, 116
  treatment of, 116
Afghan hound, hypothyroidism in, 184
Airedale, ear canal of, 6
Alaskan malamute, hypothyroidism in,
  184
  zinc-responsive dermatosis in,
    188–189
Allergen(s), definition of, 115
  exposure to, avoidance of, 116
    routes for, 115
  naturally occurring, allergic contact
    dermatitis caused by, 119
Allergic contact dermatitis (cutaneous
    drug eruption), 118–119
Allergic inhalant dermatitis. See also
    Allergy.
  ceruminous otitis with, 190–191
  clinical signs of, 190
  diagnosis of, 190
  etiology of, 190
  pathogenesis of, 190
  treatment of, 190–191
Allergy. See also *Allergic inhalant*
    dermatitis; Atopy; Fleas, allergic
    dermatitis caused by; Food
    hypersensitivity (food allergy); Otitis
    externa, allergic.
  causes of, 114–115
  diagnosis of, 190
  otitis externa caused by, 113–119
  testing for, 214

Alopecia, in flea allergy dermatitis,
  192
  in hyperadrenocorticism, 186
  in hypothyroidism, 185
American Cocker spaniel. See *Cocker
  spaniel.*
Amikacin, ototoxicity of, 147*t*
Aminoglycosides, ototoxicity of, 22, 131,
  147*t*, 150
Amitraz, for *Demodex* mites, 92, 195
Amphotericin B, ototoxicity of, 149*t*,
  151
Ampulla, *14*
Ampullary nerve, *20–21*
Anatomy, of canine and feline ear, 1–23
Anesthesia, client education about, 236
Anesthetic, topical, allergic contact
  dermatitis caused by, 119
Animax Ointment, active ingredients of,
  243
Annulus fibrocartilaginous, 9, 12
Anthelix, *2, 4, 5*
Antibacterials, active ingredients of,
  241–242
Antibiotic(s), active ingredients of,
  241–242
  aminoglycoside. See *Aminoglycosides.*
  for *Malassezia* dermatitis, 218
  for otitis externa, 104, 108, 217–218
  for otitis media, 139–140
  nonaminoglycoside, ototoxicity of, 149*t*,
    150
  ototoxicity of, 22, 108, 147*t*, 149*t*, 150
  systemic, indications for, 114, 139
  topical, indications for, 139–140
    safe, 153*t*
Antifungal agents, active ingredients of,
  242–243
  for otitis media, 140
  ototoxicity of, 149*t*, 151
Anti-inflammatory agents, for ear-canal
    stenosis, 55, *56*
  for otitis media, 139–140
  mild, active ingredients of, 241
  moderate, active ingredients of, 240
  potent, active ingredients of, 240
  topical, safe, 153*t*
Antineoplastic agents, ototoxicity of,
  147*t*
Antioxidant supplements, 216
Antiseptics, ototoxicity of, 131, 149*t*,
  150–151
Antitragus, *2, 4, 5*
Apex, of external ear, *2, 4*
Apocrine cysts, 59, *60,* 61, *61*
Apocrine gland(s). See also *Ceruminous
    gland(s).*
  of ear canal, 56–57
    in otitis externa, 59, *60,* 61, *61*
    secretion from, and ear disorders, 61

Arsenic compounds, ototoxicity of, 147*t*
Astringents, ototoxicity of, 149*t*, 152
Atopy, aeroallergy as form of, 115–116
  definition of, 115
  development of, factors affecting, 115
  diagnosis of, 190
  genetic predisposition to, 190
  in cats, 190–191
  in dogs, 190–191
  otitis externa with, 100–101, *101,* 110
    ceruminous, 190–191
  pruritus with, 214
  testing for, 214
  treatment of, 190–191, 214
Auditory canal. See *Ear canal.*
Auditory ossicles. See *Ossicles.*
Auditory tube, anatomy of, *7, 14–15,* 16,
  126
  histology of, 16
  osteum of, 16
Auricle. See *Pinna.*
Auricular artery(ies), 8
Auricular nerve(s), *9*
Auriculopalpebral nerve, *9*
Auriculotemporal nerve, *15*
Aurimite, active ingredients of, 243

B
Bacitracin, ototoxicity of, 149*t*
Bacteria. See also *Infection(s).*
  colonization of ear canal by, 47, 49, 51,
    56, 157
    in otitis externa, 106–107
  in ceruminous otitis, 182
  otitis externa caused by, culture and
    sensitivity testing in, 104,
    221–222
    cytological evaluation for, 102–104,
      103
    in hypothyroidism, 95–96
    treatment of, 61–62, 217
  otitis externa/media/interna caused by,
    magnetic resonance imaging of, in
    cat, 205–211, *207–210*
  otitis media caused by, culture and
    sensitivity testing in, 139–142
Basal cell carcinoma, of ear canal, 195
Basal keratinocytes, 156
Basilar membrane, *20–21*
Bassett hound, primary idiopathic
    seborrhea in, 183
Baytril Injection Solution, active
    ingredients of, 243
  for otitis externa, 108
  for otitis media, 139
Beck curette, 40
Benzalkonium chloride, ototoxicity of,
  149*t*, 151

Benzethonium chloride, ototoxicity of, 149t, 151
Betamethasone, products containing, 240
Bleeding, during flushing of tympanic bulla, 138
  from ear, 64, 64
Bleomycin, ototoxicity of, 147t
Blood vessels, auricular, 2, 4, 5, 8
Boxer, hypothyroidism in, 184
Bruising, in hyperadrenocorticism, 186
Buccal nerve(s), 9, 15
Bulla tympanica. See Tympanic bulla.
Bumetanide, ototoxicity of, 147t
Bur-O-Cort 2:1, active ingredients of, 243
Burotic hc, active ingredients of, 244

C
Calcification, of ear canal, 51, 53, 132, 134
Canalography, 125
Candida albicans, in ear canal, in otitis externa, 107
Carbamide peroxide, ototoxicity of, 149t
Carbenicillin, as safe ototopical agent, 153t
Carboplatin, ototoxicity of, 147t
Carcinoma of undetermined origin, of ear canal, in cats, 75
  in dogs, 75
Carotid canal, 10, 12–14, 14
Carotid plexus, 13–14
Carrier vehicles, ototoxicity of, 149t, 152
Cartilage(s), annular, anatomy of, 2, 2–3, 6, 7, 10
  auricular, anatomy of, 2, 2–3, 10
    breed-specific shape and size of, 4
    hematoma of, 8
    skin covering of, 4
    thickening of, 51–54
    tubus auris of, 5, 5
    vasculature of, 2, 4
  conchal, 7
  of external ear, 2, 2–3, 3
  scutiform, anatomy of, 2, 2–3, 3, 6
    functions of, 3, 6
Cat(s), allergic dermatitis in, 189
  allergic inhalant dermatitis in, 190–191
  bacterial otitis externa/media/interna in, magnetic resonance imaging of, 205–211, 207–210
  ceruminous gland tumors in, 71–72, 75, 195
  computed tomography of, 202, 203–204
  ear canal of, ventilation of, 6, 46
  ear mites in, 90. See also Ear mites.
  ear of, anatomy of, 1–23
  ear-canal tumors in. See also Tumor(s).
    benign, 75, 195
      ceruminous otitis with, 195–196
      incidence of, 75

Cat(s) (Continued)
    malignant, 75, 195
  external ear of. See External ear.
  fatty acid deficiency in, 187
  fleas on, and ear symptoms, 92, 93
  food hypersensitivity in, 191–192
  hypothyroidism in, 184
  inflammatory polyps in. See Inflammatory polyps.
  inner ear of, 17
  magnetic resonance imaging in, 205–211, 206–210
  middle ear cavity of, 16, 17
    bony septum of, 16, 17
    nerves of, 16, 18
  nasopharyngeal polyps in, 80–81, 195–196. See also Inflammatory polyps.
  open-mouth rostro-occipital radiograph of, 71, 133
  otitis media in, primary, 107
  sarcoptic mite of, ceruminous otitis caused by, 194
  sebaceous gland adenocarcinoma in, 75
  soft wax ball in, 161–164
  squamous cell carcinoma of tympanum in, computed tomography of, 202, 203–204
  tympanic membrane of, otoscopic appearance of, 31, 32
    perforation of, 66
    rupture of, 171–173, 172
  vitamin A metabolism in, 188
  white, with congenital deafness, 22–23
Cava conchae, 5
  innervation of, 8
Cefmenoxime, as safe ototopical agent, 153t
Ceftazidime, as safe ototopical agent, 153t
Cephalexin, for pyoderma, 217
Cerumen, 7–8, 182
  clearance of, in ear canal, 58–59, 156–157
  components of, 57–58
  concretions of. See Ceruminoliths.
  dry, 57–58, 58
  functions of, 58
  impaction of, 58
  otoscopic appearance of, 26, 27
  production of, 57
    excessive, and otitis externa, 56–62, 57, 60
  removal of, 58–59
    ear flushes for, 61–62
  soft plug of, 158, 159
  tumors obscured by, 68, 69
  wet, 57–58, 59
Ceruminoliths, 59, 60, 159, 159
  clinical signs of, 160, 161
  detection of, 159

Ceruminoliths *(Continued)*
  formation of, 159–160
  hair included in, 159–160, *160*
  otoscopic examination of, 160
  removal of, 161–164, *162–164*
Ceruminolytic agent(s), 161
  ototoxicity of, 149*t,* 151–152
  safe, 153*t*
Ceruminous gland(s), adenocarcinoma of,
    71–72
  in cats, 75, 195
  in dogs, 75, 195
  incidence of, 75
  adenomas of, *49*
    ear canal occlusion by, 54, *54*
    gross examination of, 72, *73*
    in cats, 75, 195
    in dogs, 195
    incidence of, 75
    ulcerated, *70*
  carcinoma of, in cats, 195
  cystic, 59, *60,* 61, *61,* 182
  hyperplasia of, 195–196
  of ear canal, 7, 57, *57,* 182
CERUMITE, active ingredients of, 244
Cervical ganglion, superior, 13–14
Cervicoauricularis superficialis muscle, *3*
Cervicoscutularis muscle, *3*
Cetrimide, ototoxicity of, 149*t*
Cheyletiella, ceruminous otitis caused by,
    195
Chinese Shar Pei. See *Shar Pei.*
Chloramphenicol, antibacterials
    containing, 241
  ototoxicity of, 149*t*
Chlora-Otic, active ingredients of, 244
Chlorhexidine, ototoxicity of, 149*t,* 151
Chloromycetin Otic, active ingredients of,
    244
Chloroquine, ototoxicity of, 147*t*
Chlortetracycline, ototoxicity of, 149*t*
Cholesteatoma, acquired, 127
  congenital, 127, *128*
  definition of, 127
  pathogenesis of, 127–129
Chondrosarcoma, of ear canal, 195
Chorda tympani, *14–15,* 18, *19,* 126
Chow chow, hypothyroidism in, 95, 184
Cipro HC Otic, active ingredients of, 244
Ciprofloxacin, antibacterials containing,
    241
  as safe ototopical agent, 153*t*
Cisplatin, ototoxicity of, 147*t*
Cleaning agent(s), 219–220
  ototoxicity of, 149*t,* 151–152
Clear X Ear Drying Solution, active
    ingredients of, 244
Clotrimazole, antifungals containing, 242
  as safe ototopical agent, 153*t*

Cochlea, anatomy of, *14,* 16, *19,* 20, *20–21,*
    22–23
  functions of, 22
  ototoxins and, 131
  spiral ganglion of, *20–21*
Cochlear aqueduct, *14,* 16, 20
Cochlear duct, *20–21,* 22
Cochlear nerve, *19,* 20, *20–21,* 22
Cochlear promontory, 7, 12, *13–15,* 16, *19*
Cochlear (round) window, 12, *13–15,* 16, *19*
  damage to, and ototoxicity, 131
Cocker spaniel, cerumen gland adenoma
    in, *73*
  Demodex mites in, *93*
  ear canal of, calcification of, *53,* 132, *134*
    stenosis of, *53,* 54, *54*
  ear-canal tumor in, *70*
  hypothyroidism in, 95, 184
  primary idiopathic seborrhea in,
      183–184, 216
  stenotic ear canal in, *48*
  vitamin A–responsive dermatosis in, 188
Colistin, antibacterials containing, 241
  ototoxicity of, 149*t*
Collagen, of tympanic membrane, 126, *126*
Collie, tympanic bulla of, flushing solution
    in, radiographic appearance of, *135*
Coly-Mycin S Otic, active ingredients of,
    244
Comedones, in hyperadrenocorticism, 186
Compliance issues, in home treatment,
    233
Computed tomography (CT), 198–202
  advantages and disadvantages of, 198,
      205, 211
  applications of, 132, 198
  of cat, 202, *203–204*
  of dog, *199–201,* 199–202
  of middle-ear tumor, 68
  of tympanic bullae, 132
  principles of, 198
  sensitivity of disease detection using,
      198–199
Conofite Lotion, active ingredients of, 244
Corpus adiposum auriculae, 6
CORT/ASTRIN Solution, active
    ingredients of, 244
Corticosteroids, anti-inflammatory effects
    of, in stenosis of ear canal, 55, *56*
  contraindications to, 114
  for ear mite hypersensitivity, in cats, 90
  for food allergy, 117
  for inflammatory polyps, in follow-up
      therapy, 85
  for otitis externa, 107–108
  for otitis media, 139
  for pruritus, 217, 220
  hyperadrenocorticism caused by, 186
Cortisol, serum, excess, 185–186

German shepherd *(Continued)*
  otitis externa in, perpetuating factors in, 107
  primary idiopathic seborrhea in, 183
  ruptured eardrum in, *137, 170*
German shorthaired pointer, zinc-responsive dermatosis in, 189
Glycerin, ototoxicity of, 152
Gold salts, ototoxicity of, 147*t*
Golden retriever, ceruminous gland tumor in, *76–77*
  ear-canal tumor in, *70*
  hypothyroidism in, 95, 184
Gramicidin, ototoxicity of, 149*t*
Great Dane, hypothyroidism in, 184
  zinc-responsive dermatosis in, 188–189
Griseofulvin, ototoxicity of, 149*t*

H
Hair, in ear canal, 6, 26, *27–28,* 29, 50, *135*
  and ceruminoliths, 159–160, *160*
  and otitis externa, 55–56, 111
  loss of, in otitis externa, 32, 111
  removal of, 56
  regrowth of, in hyperadrenocorticism, 186
Hair cells, 22
  ototoxin and, 131
  outer, *20–21*
Hearing, air conduction, 123
  bone conduction, 123
  deficit. See also *Deafness.*
    with otitis media, 123
Helicotrema, *14,* 22
Helix, distal crus of (spine), *2, 4*
  lateral border of, *2*
  lateral crus of, *2, 4*
  medial border of, *2*
  medial crus of, *2, 4*
Hemangiosarcoma, of ear canal, in dogs, 75
Hematoma(s), aural, 8
  recurrent, *70*
Histiocytoma, of ear canal, in dogs, 75
Home treatment, compliance issues in, 233
Hormonal hypersensitivity, 118
Horner's syndrome, 18, 122, 138
Hydrocortisone, products containing, 241
Hydrocortisone acetate, products containing, 241
Hygromycin B, ototoxicity of, 149*t*
Hyperadrenocorticism, causes of, 185–186
  ceruminous otitis in, 185–186
  diagnosis of, 186
  treatment of, 186
Hyperandrogenism, in male dogs, ceruminous otitis with, 186

Hyperpigmentation, in hypothyroidism, 185
Hypersensitivity reaction(s). See also *Food hypersensitivity (food allergy).*
  common types of, 115, 189
  delayed, 115, 117–118
  immediate, 115, 117
  pruritus with, 214
  to ear mites, 88, 90, 193
Hypoglossal canal, *13*
Hypoglossus muscle, *7*
Hypothyroidism, and
  hyperadrenocorticism, combination of, 186
  in cats, 184
  in dogs, ceruminous otitis in, 184–185
    clinical signs of, 185
    congenital, 184
    dermatologic abnormalities in, 185
    diagnosis of, 185
    ear disorders caused by, 94–96, 110, 184–185
    etiology of, 184
    primary, 184
    seborrheic dermatitis in, 95
    secondary, 184
    thyroglobulin assays in, 94–95
    treatment of, 185

I
Imaging. See also *Radiography.*
  advanced techniques of, 197–211. See also *Computed tomography (CT); Magnetic resonance imaging (MR).*
Immunoglobulin E, in hypersensitivity, 115
Immunoglobulin G, in hypersensitivity, 115
Immunotherapy, 116
Incisure, antitragohelicine, *2*
  intertragic, *2, 4*
  lateral, *2*
  pretragic, *2, 4*
Incus, 13, *14–15*
  anatomy of, 14–15
Infection(s). See also *Pyoderma.*
  epithelial damage caused by, 157
  external ear. See *Otitis externa.*
  middle ear. See *Otitis media.*
  secondary, with allergic inhalant dermatitis, 190–191
    with ceruminous otitis, 183–184
    with *Demodex* mite infestation, 194
    with ear mite infestation, 90, 193
    with ear-canal tumors, 195–196
    with fatty acid deficiency, 187–188
    with flea allergy dermatitis, 192

Infection(s) *(Continued)*
  with hyperadrenocorticism, 186
  with hypothyroidism, 95–96, 110, 185
  with otitis externa, 106–107, 196
  with tumor, 68–72, *70*
  with vitamin A deficiency, 188
  with zinc-responsive dermatosis, 189
  specimens in, cytological examination of,
      40–41, *42–43*
  treatment of, 217–218
  steroid-free approach to, 114, 118
Inflammatory polyps, in cats, clinical signs
      of, 80–81
  ear mites and, 90
  eardrum rupture caused by, 171–173,
      172
  follow-up therapy for, 85
  histology of, 82
  histopathology of, 195
  incidence of, 80
  localization of, 80
  origin of, 80
  otitis externa related to, 81, 85, 195
  otitis media related to, 80–81, 85
  otoscopic appearance of, 80–81, *82*
  pathogenesis of, 81–82
  pedunculated, 83, *83*
  recurrence of, 85
  removal of, 83–85, *84–85*
  waxy accumulations with, 80, *80,* 195
  in dogs, 83, *83,* 85, *86,* 195
Inner ear, anatomy of, *14, 19, 20–21,* 20–23
  feline, *17*
  functions of, 20
  injury, by ototoxic agents, 146
  innervation of, 20, *20–21*
  penetration of topical agents into,
      factors affecting, 146–148
Insecticide, allergic contact dermatitis
      caused by, 119
Internal auricular nerve(s), 8–9, *9*
Internal carotid artery, 18
Internal carotid nerves, *15,* 18
Interparietoscutularis muscle, *3*
Interscutularis muscle, *3*
Interstitial cell tumor, ceruminous otitis
      with, 186
Iodine, ototoxicity of, 149*t,* 151
Iodochlorhydroxyquinolone, ototoxicity of,
      149*t*
Iodophors, ototoxicity of, 149*t,* 151
Irish setter, primary idiopathic seborrhea
      in, 183
Isoflupredone acetate, products containing,
      240
Isopropyl myristate, as safe ototopical
      agent, 153*t*
Itraconazole, for *Malassezia* dermatitis, 218
  for otitis media, 140

Ivermectin, extra-label use of, 218
  for *Demodex* mites, 195
  for ear mites, 91–92, 220
  for parasitic infestations, 218
  injectable, products containing, 243
  injections of, adverse reactions to, 92
      indications for, 92
Ivomec 1% Injection for Cattle and Swine,
      active ingredients of, 246

K
Kanamycin, ototoxicity of, 131, 147*t*
Keratinization disorders, 215. See also
      Seborrhea.
  ceruminous otitis in, 183–186
  ear disorders caused by, 94–96
Keratinocytes, barrier functions of, 157
  basal, 156
  immune functions of, 157
Keratoconjunctivitis sicca, 122
Ketoconazole, for *Malassezia* dermatitis,
      218
  for otitis media, 140

L
Labrador retriever, chronic ear infections
      in, imaging of, *199–201,* 199–202
  management of, 202
  inflammatory polyps in, *86*
  middle ear tumor in, *77*
  otitis media in, radiographic assessment
      of, *135*
  vitamin A–responsive dermatosis in,
      188
  zinc-responsive dermatosis in, 189
Labyrinth, membranous, 20, *20–21,* 22.
      See also *Cochlea; Semicircular
      canal(s); Vestibule.*
  problems in, 22
  osseous, *10,* 20
  anatomy of, *10,* 20–22
Limbus, of tympanic membrane, *19*
Lingual nerve, *15*
Liquichlor, active ingredients of, 246
Lotrisone, active ingredients of, 246
Lymphocytic thyroiditis, in dogs,
      hypothyroidism caused by, 94–95, 184
Lymphoma, of middle ear, 75

M
Magnetic resonance imaging (MR),
      advantages and disadvantages of, 198,
      205, 211

Magnetic resonance imaging (MR)
 (Continued)
 applications of, 198, 205
 in cats, 205–211, *206–210*
 principles of, 202–205
 sensitivity of disease detection using,
  199
Malassezia, colonization of ear canal, in
  otitis externa, *42–43,* 107, 182
 dermatitis caused by, *100*
  treatment of, 218–219
 infection by, ear involvement in, *100*
  in allergic inhalant dermatitis,
   190–191
  in *Demodex* mite infestation, 194
  in ear mite infestation, 193
  in fatty acid deficiency, 187–188
  in flea allergy dermatitis, 192
  in hyperadrenocorticism, 186
  in hypothyroidism, 95, 110
  in neoplasia, 195–196
  in vitamin A deficiency, 188
  in zinc-responsive dermatosis, 189
  secondary, with ceruminous otitis,
   183–184
 otitis externa caused by, *65*
  cytological evaluation for, 102–104,
   103
  ear cleaning in, 219–220
  treatment of, 109–110, 218–219
Malleus, 13, *14–15,* 126
 anatomy of, 14–16
 footplate of, otoscopic appearance of, *30*
 manubrium of, 10–11, *11,* 12, 14–15, *19*
  otoscopic appearance of, 29–30, *64*
 otoscopic appearance of, 29–30, *39*
Mandibular fossa, *13*
Mannitol, ototoxicity of, 147*t*
Manubrium of malleus, 10–11, *11,* 12,
  14–15, *19*
 otoscopic appearance of, 29–30, *64*
Marginal pouch, of pinna, 4, *4*
Marketing, client reminders in, 234–235
 communication and, 227
 convenience and, 233
 creativity in, 235–236
 definition of, 225
 enthusiasm and, 227–228
 follow-up and, 235
 fundamentals of, 225–226
 of ear care and otitis therapy, 223–237
 perceptions and, 226–227
 staff's role in, 229
 strategies for, 228–236
 successful, elements of, 227
 trust and, 226
Masseteric nerve, *15*
Mast cell tumor, of ear canal, 195
Mechlorethamine, ototoxicity of, 147*t*

Medication(s), active ingredients of,
  functions of, 240–243
 listed by product trade name, 243–249
 allergic contact dermatitis caused by,
  118–119
 concretions of, in ear canal, 96, *96*
 improper use of, otitis externa caused by,
  196
 systemic, ototoxicity of, 146, 147*t*
 topical, ototoxicity of, 146–148, 149*t*
Melanoma, in dogs, benign, 75
 malignant, 75
Mercury, ototoxicity of, 149*t*
Merthiolate, ototoxicity of, 149*t,* 151
Miconazole, antifungals containing, 242
Miconazole Lotion 1%, active ingredients
  of, 247
Miconazole Lotion 1%, active ingredients
  of, 247
Middle ear, anatomy of, 12–20, *28*
 canine, nerves of, *15,* 18, *19*
 cavity of, *10*
  in cats, 16, *17*
  in dogs, *15,* 18, *19*
  nerves in relation to, 13–14, *15*
 ear mites in, 90
 false, 30–32, 127
 feline, 16, *17*
  bony septum of, 16, *17*
  nerves of, 16, 18
 flushing and vacuuming of, 136–138,
  137–138
 inflammatory polyps in, 80
 injury, by ototoxic agents, 146
 nerves of, *14–15,* 16, 18–19, *19*
  iatrogenic injury to, 138
  in transit, 18
 penetration of topical agents into,
  factors affecting, 146–148
 polyp of, 68, *71*
 tumors of, 68, *71,* 75
Milbemycin oxime, for *Demodex* mites,
  195
Miniature schnauzer, vitamin
  A–responsive dermatosis in, 188
Minocycline, ototoxicity of, 149*t*
Miosis, definition of, 18
Mita-Clear, active ingredients of, 247
MITAPLEX-R, active ingredients of,
  247
Mites. See *Demodex mites; Ear mites;*
  Otobius megnini; Sarcoptes scabiei.
Miticidals, active ingredients of, 243
Modiolus, *19,* 22
 lamina of, *19*
Mucoperiosteum, in otitis externa, 106
 in otitis media, 177
Musculotubal canal, *13*
Mylohyoid nerve, *15*

Mylohyoideus muscle, 7
Myringotomy, *39,* 39–40, 171
  iatrogenic, 171
  in diagnosis of otitis media, 140–142
  traumatic, 65, *66,* 67, *67,* 170–171, *171*
Myxedema, in hypothyroidism, 185

N
Nasopharynx, inflammatory polyps in, 123
  eardrum rupture caused by, 171–173,
    172
  imaging of, *134,* 199
  in cats, 80–81, *134,* 195–196
Neomycin, allergic contact dermatitis
    caused by, 119
  antibacterials containing, 241–242
  contact dermatitis caused by, in ear
    canal, 55
  ototoxicity of, 131
  precautions with, 108
Neoplasia, of ear canals, 67–78. See also
    Tumor(s).
Neo-Predef, active ingredients of, 247
Netilmicin, ototoxicity of, 147*t*
Newfoundland hound, hypothyroidism in,
    184
Nolvamite, active ingredients of, 247
Notoedres cati, ceruminous otitis caused
    by, 194
Nutritional deficiency, ceruminous otitis
    with, 187–189
Nystatin, antifungals containing, 242
  as safe ototopical agent, 153*t*

O
Occipital condyle, *13*
Occipitalis muscle, *3*
Ofloxacin, antibacterials containing, 242
  as safe ototopical agent, 153*t*
  for otitis externa, 108, 140
  for otitis media, 140
Old English sheepdog, ear canal of, 6
  external acoustic meatus in, stenosis of,
    50
Organ of Corti. See *Spiral organ.*
Oropharynx, inflammatory polyps in, in
    cats, 80–81
Ossicles, *28*
  amplification of sound waves by, 15
  anatomy of, *14,* 14–16, 126
  skeletal muscles associated with, *14,* 16
Otic ganglion, *15,* 19
Otic nerve, *28*
Oticare-M Ear Mite Treatment, active
    ingredients of, 247

Otitis, client education about, 231–233
  noninfectious causes of, 195–196
  microscopic findings in, 41, *42*
  pruritic. See also *Pruritus.*
    clinical treatment trial for, 215–219
    complications of, management of, 221
    culture and sensitivity testing in,
      221–222
    ear cleaning in, 219–220
    ear therapy in, protocol for, 219–222
    surgery in, 222
    systemic therapy for, 221
    topical therapy for, 220–221
    treatment of, 214
  treatment of, marketing of, 223–237
Otitis externa, allergic, 113–119
  in cutaneous drug eruption, 118–119
  in food hypersensitivity, 117–118
  in hormonal hypersensitivity, 118
  atopy and, 100–101, *101,* 110, 190–191
  bacterial, culture and sensitivity testing
    in, 104, 221–222
  cytological evaluation for, 102–104,
    103
  in hypothyroidism, 95–96, 110
  magnetic resonance imaging of, in cat,
    205–211, *207–210*
  treatment of, 61–62, 104, 219–222
  ceruminous, *33,* 56–62, *57, 60,* 181–196
    clinical signs of, 183–184
    conformational causes of, 196
    definition of, 182
    Demodex mites and, 194–195
    ear-canal tumors and, 195–196
    environmental causes of, 196
    etiology of, 182
    in allergic dermatitis, 189–192
    in allergic inhalant dermatitis,
      190–191
    in atopy, 190–191
    in ear mite infestation, 192–193
    in endocrine dermatosis, 184–186
    in fatty acid deficiency, 187–188
    in flea allergy dermatitis, 192
    in food hypersensitivity, 191–192
    in hyperadrenocorticism, 185–186
    in hypothyroidism, 95, 184–185
    in keratinization disorders, 183–186
    in nutritional deficiency, 187–189
    in parasitic dermatosis, 192–195
    in primary idiopathic seborrhea,
      183–184
    in vitamin A–responsive dermatosis,
      188
    in zinc-responsive dermatosis,
      188–189
    Notoedres cati and, 194
    Otobius megnini and, 194
    Sarcoptes scabiei and, 193–194

Otitis externa *(Continued)*
  chronic, clinical characteristics of,
    105–106, *106*
    epithelial hyperplasia in, 51, *51–52*
    pathophysiology of, 6
  cytological evaluation in, 102–104,
    103
  dermatological conditions and, *100,*
    100–101, *101,* 104
  ear-canal examination in, 105–106
  eardrum rupture in, 129, *129*
  exudates in, 101, *101,* 106, 129–130
  follow-up therapy for, 110–111
  hair in ear canal and, 55–56, 111
  hair loss in, 32, 111
  in cats, incidence of, 100
  in dogs, breeds predisposed to, 59
    incidence of, 100
  in hypothyroidism, 95–96, 110
  infections secondary to, 106–107
  inflammatory polyps and, 81
  Malassezia, 100, 102–104, *103*
  microbiology of, 102–104, *103,* 106–107
  microscopic findings in, 41, *42–43,*
    102–104, *103*
  otitis media secondary to, 107, 129–130,
    170
  otoscopic findings in, *33*
  overtreatment of ears and, 55
  pathogenesis of, 47
  pathology of, 105–106
  perpetuating factors in, 106–107
    management of, 111
  predisposing factors for, definition of, 46
    treatment of, 46, 130
    types of, 46–47
  resolution of, signs of, 111
  secondary to ear mites, 104
    treatment of, 92
  stenotic ear canal and, *48,* 49, *49*
  treatment of, 100, 107–110, 130
    flushing of ear canal in, 104–105
    new approaches to, 101–102
    ototoxic agents used in, 148, 149*t*
  tumors and, 68, *70,* 104
  yeast, cytological evaluation for, 102–104
    treatment of, 61–62
Otitis interna, bacterial, magnetic
    resonance imaging of, in cat, 205–211,
    207–210
Otitis media, acute, 122
  prevention of, 130
  bacterial, culture and sensitivity testing
    in, 139–142
    magnetic resonance imaging of, in cat,
      205–211, *207–210*
  chronic, 140
    eardrum rupture in, 37, *37*
    facial nerve involvement in, 18

Otitis media *(Continued)*
    permanent, 177, *177*
    spread of, 20–22
  clinical signs of, 122–123
  eardrum examination in, 123–125
  eardrum healing in, 138, 140, *141,*
    141–142, 174–178, *175–176*
  eardrum rupture in, 129–130
  exudates in, 129–130, *130,* 132, *135*
  fungal, treatment of, 140
  healed eardrum and, 123, *124,* 138, 140,
    141
  hearing deficit with, 123, 138
  history with, 122–123
  iatrogenic, 67
  imaging of, 198–199
  in cats, prevalence of, 107
  in dogs, prevalence of, 107
  inflammatory polyps and, 80–81
  microbiology of, 107
  otorrhea with, 122
  otoscopic findings in, *37,* 37–38,
    122–123, *124,* 136–138, *137–138*
  ototoxins and, 131
  pathogenesis of, 122, 127
  pathophysiology of, 122, 132
  plant awns and, 97
  prevalence of, 123
  primary, 107
  radiographic evaluation in, 131–132,
    133–135
  resolution of, 140, *141*
  secondary to otitis externa, 107, 170
  suppurative, eardrum rupture caused
    by, 171
  treatment of, 132–140
    anti-inflammatory measures in,
      139–140
    flushing of tympanic bulla in,
      136–138, *137–138*
    surgical approach for, 142
    yeast, treatment of, 140
Otobius megnini, ceruminous otitis caused
    by, 194
Otodectes cyanotis. See *Ear mites.*
Otomax, active ingredients of, 247
Otomite Plus, active ingredients of, 247
Otorrhea, with otitis media, 122
Otoscope, videographic, 33–37, *34, 36*
  advantages of, 230
  ceruminolith removal using, 161, *163*
  documentation capability of, 35–37
  ear mite visualization using, 88
  eardrum rupture diagnosis using,
    125
  foreign body removal using, 97
  in staff education, 229
  inflammatory polyp removal using,
    83–85, *84*

Otoscope *(Continued)*
inflammatory polyp visualization using, 81, *82*
tumor removal using, 78
tumor visualization using, 68
tympanic membrane suctioning using, 136–138, *137*
Otoscopy, 26
ear mite visualization using, 88
evaluation of ear canal using, 32
indications for, 196
Ototopical agents, allergic contact dermatitis caused by, 118–119
for pruritic otitis, 220–221
ototoxicity of, 131, 146, 149*t*
factors affecting, 146–148
safe, 152–153, 153*t*
steroid-free, 114
tympanic membrane perforation and, 131, 146, 148–153
Ototoxicity, clinical signs of, 146–148
definition of, 146
development of, factors affecting, 146–148
of systemic agents, 146, 147*t*
of topical agents, 131, 146, 149*t*
factors affecting, 146–148
precautions against, 131, 153
Oval window. See *Vestibular (oval) window.*
Oxytetracycline, ototoxicity of, 149*t*

P
Palpebral nerve, *9*
Panalog Ointment, active ingredients of, 247
Papilloma, of ear canal, in cats, 75
in dogs, 75
Parasites, dermatosis caused by, ceruminous otitis with, 192–195
treatment of, 218
ear disorders caused by, 88–94, 104. See also *Demodex mites; Ear mites; Fleas; Ticks.*
Parasiticides, ototoxicity of, 149*t*, 152
Parotidoauricularis muscle, 7
Pars flaccida, of tympanic membrane, 9–10, *11*, 173, *173*
otoscopic appearance of, 30, *30–31*
Pars tensa, of tympanic membrane, 9–11, *11*, *19*
otoscopic appearance of, 29, *30*
Penicillin G, as safe ototopical agent, 153*t*
Pentobarbital, ototoxicity of, 147*t*
Perilymph fluid, 15–16, 20
Persian cat, apocrine cysts in, *60*
Petrobasilar fissure. See *Tympano-occipital fissure.*
Petro-occipital canal. See *Carotid canal.*

Petro-occipital fissure. See *Tympano-occipital fissure.*
Petrosal nerve, major, *15*
minor, *15*, 19
Petrosal venous sinus, ventral, *10*, 14
Petrous temporal bone, 126
pyramidal part of, 20
cerebellar surface of, 20
cerebral surface of, 20
Pharmacetin, ototoxicity of, 149*t*
Pinna, *28*
anatomy of, 3–6, *4*
carriage of, in cats, 3
in dogs, 3
in fatty acid deficiency, 187
innervation of, 8–9, *9*
lateral (caudal) margin of, *2*, 3–4, *4*
marginal pouch of, 4, *4*
medial (rostral) margin of, *2*, 3–4, *4*
seborrheic, in hypothyroidism, 185
traction on, for straightening ear canal, 26
trauma to, 62–67
vasculature of, 8
Plant awns, in ear canal, 96–97, *97*
Plasmacytoma, of ear canal, in dogs, 75
Polyethylene glycol, ototoxicity of, 149*t*, 152
Polymyxin B, ototoxicity of, 149*t*
Polymyxin B sulfate, antibacterials containing, 242
Polyp(s), inflammatory. See *Inflammatory polyps.*
nasopharyngeal, *71*, 123, 195–196. See also *Inflammatory polyps.*
eardrum rupture caused by, 171–173, *172*
imaging of, *134*, 199
of ear canal, in cats, 75
in dogs, 75
of middle ear, 68, *71*
oropharyngeal, in cats, 81. See also *Inflammatory polyps.*
Poodle, ceruminolith in, *159*
ear canal of, hair in, *27*
eardrum perforation in, *137*
hypothyroidism in, 95
iatrogenic myringotomy in, *67*
stenotic ear canal in, *48*
zinc-responsive dermatosis in, 189
Potassium bromide, ototoxicity of, 147*t*, 149*t*
Practice issues. See *Ear care services; Marketing.*
Prednisolone, for otitis externa, 108
products containing, 241
Pressure tympanometry, 125
Pricing, of ear care services, 233–234
Professional practice. See *Ear care services; Marketing.*
Propylene glycol, ototoxicity of, 149*t*, 152

Proteus, colonization of ear canal, in otitis
    externa, 107, 182
    otitis externa caused by, 102, *103*
    otitis media caused by, 139
Pruritus, aeroallergy and, 116
    atopy and, 214
    clinical treatment trial for, 215–218
        results of, analysis of, 218–219
    cutaneous drug eruption and, 118–119
    flea allergy and, 192, 214
    food allergy and, 214
    hypersensitivity reactions and, 214
    persistent, 218–219
    treatment of, 214
Pseudomonas, chronic ear infection caused
        by, *199–201,* 199–202
    colonization of ear canal of, in otitis
        externa, 107, 182
    otitis externa caused by, *101,* 102, *103*
        and tympanic membrane healing, *176*
        treatment of, 108–109, 220, 222
    otitis media caused by, 107, 139, 222
        and tympanic membrane healing, *176*
Ptosis, definition of, 18
Pyoderma, in hyperadrenocorticism, 186
    in hypothyroidism, 185
    treatment of, 217
Pyrethrins, products containing, 243

Q
Q-tips. See *Cotton-tipped applicators.*
Quadritop Ointment, active ingredients of,
    247
Quinidine, ototoxicity of, 147*t*
Quinine, ototoxicity of, 147*t*

R
Radiation therapy, for tumors of ear canal,
    78
Radiography. See also *Imaging.*
    contrast, in facial wounds, *63*
        in tympanic membrane rupture, 125
    in otitis media, 131–132
    of middle-ear tumor, 68, *71*
Respiratory infection, eardrum rupture
        caused by, 171, *172*
Retro-articular foramen, *13, 15*
Retro-articular process, *19*
Ribostamycin, ototoxicity of, 147*t*
Ristocetin, ototoxicity of, 147*t*
Rotenone, and cube resins, products
        containing, 243
    products containing, 243
Round cell tumor, of ear canal, in dogs, 75
Round window. See *Cochlear (round)
    window.*

S
Saccular nerve, *20–21*
Saccule, *14,* 22
Salicylates, ototoxicity of, 147*t*
Salivary gland(s), innervation of, 18–19
    mandibular, *7*
    parotid, 5, *5, 7, 10*
Sarcoma, of ear canal, in dogs, 75
Sarcoptes scabiei, ceruminous otitis caused
        by, 193–194
    treatment of, 218–219
Scabies. See *Sarcoptes scabiei.*
Scala media, *20–21,* 22
Scala tympani, 12, *14, 19, 20–21,* 22
Scala vestibuli, *19, 20–21,* 22
Scapha, *2, 4*
Schnauzer, ear-canal tumor in, *69*
Scutoauricularis superficialis dorsalis
        muscle, *3*
Sebaceous gland(s), adenocarcinoma of, in
        cats, 75, 195
    in dogs, 195
    adenomas of, in cats, 195
    in dogs, 75, 195
    hyperactivity of, 182
    hyperplasia of, 51, *52,* 182
    of ear canal, 7, 56–57, 182
Seborrhea, in allergic inhalant dermatitis,
        190
    in hyperadrenocorticism, 186
    in hypothyroidism, 185
    primary idiopathic, ceruminous otitis in,
        183–184
        diagnosis of, 184
        pathophysiology of, 183, 216
        treatment of, 184
    treatment of, 215–216
Seborrhea oleosa, 215–216
Seborrhea sicca, 215
Seborrheic dermatitis, in hypothyroidism,
        95, 185
Sedation, client education about, 236
Semicircular canal(s), *14,* 16, 20
Seminoma, ceruminous otitis with, 186
Sertoli cell tumor, ceruminous otitis with,
        186
Shampoo, acetic acid–boric acid
        (MalAcetic), bathing procedure using,
        216
    for *Malassezia* dermatitis, 218
Shampoo therapy, for pruritus, 215–216
Shar Pei, ear canal of, 50–51
    hypothyroidism in, 95, 184
    primary idiopathic seborrhea in,
        183
Sheltie, otitis media in, and tympanic
        membrane healing, *175*
Shetland sheepdog, ear canal of, stenosis
        of, *52*
    healed eardrum in, *141*

Shih Tzu, otitis media in, and tympanic membrane healing, *176*
Siberian husky, zinc-responsive dermatosis in, 188–189
Silvadene Creme 1%, active ingredients of, 248
Silver sulfadiazine, allergic contact dermatitis caused by, 119
 antibacterials containing, 242
 cream, for otitis externa, 108–109
Sisomicin, ototoxicity of, 147*t*
Skin, diseases of, ear involvement in, 41–43
 in allergic inhalant dermatitis, 190
 in cutaneous drug eruption, 118–119
 in fatty acid deficiency, 187
 in flea allergy dermatitis, 192
 in hyperadrenocorticism, 186
 in hypothyroidism, 185
 in vitamin A deficiency, 188
Sneezing, eardrum rupture caused by, in cats, 171, *172*
Solvent(s), ototoxicity of, 149*t*, 151–152
 safe, 153*t*
Spiral ganglion, of cochlea, *20–21*
Spiral lamina, osseous (bony), *19,* 22
 secondary, *19*
Spiral organ, *20–21,* 22
Springer spaniel, lichenoid-psoriasiform dermatosis of, 183
 primary idiopathic seborrhea in, 183
Squalene, as safe ototopical agent, 153*t*
Squamous cell carcinoma, of ear canal, in cats, 75
 in dogs, 75
 of osseous bullae and soft tissue, magnetic resonance imaging of, in cat, 205, *206*
 of tympanum, computed tomography of, in cat, 202, *203–204*
Stapedius muscle, 13, *14,* 16
 innervation of, 19
Stapes, 12–13, *14–15*
 anatomy of, 14–15
Staphylococcus, colonization of ear canal by, in otitis externa, 107
 otitis externa caused by, *33,* 102–104
 treatment of, 108
 otitis media caused by, treatment of, 139
Steroids. See *Corticosteroids.*
Streptococci, β-hemolytic, in otitis media, 107
Streptomycin, ototoxicity of, 147*t*
Stria mallearis, 11, *11*
Stria vascularis, *20–21*
Striae, in hyperadrenocorticism, 186
Stridor, 123
Styloid process, *2*
Stylomastoid foramen, *13*

Subarachnoid space, *14,* 20
Surgery, for otitis media, 142
 in ear canal, for pruritic otitis, 222
 for stenosis, 55
 for tumors, 75–78
 postoperative complications of, 62–64
 trauma caused by, 62–64
Synotic Otic Solution. See also *Fluocinolone.*
 active ingredients of, 248
 for otitis media, 139

T
Tailfold pyoderma, in English bulldog, 46
Tar(s), allergic contact dermatitis caused by, 119
Taste buds, innervation of, 18
Tectorial membrane, *20–21,* 22
Temporal bone, petrosal part of, 20. See also *Petrous temporal bone.*
Tensor tympani muscle, 13, *14,* 16
 innervation of, *15,* 19
Tetracycline, ototoxicity of, 149*t*
Thiabendazole, products containing, 243
Thyroglobulin assays, in hypothyroidism, 94–95
Thyroid gland, disorders of. See also *Hypothyroidism.*
 in dogs, 184
Thyroid hormone(s), actions of, 185
 deficiency of. See *Hypothyroidism.*
 levels of, in thyroidal versus nonthyroidal illness, 95
Thyroid stimulation test, indications for, 185–186
Thyroid-stimulating hormone, levels of, in thyroidal versus nonthyroidal illness, 95
Thyroxine, levels of, in thyroidal versus nonthyroidal illness, 95
Ticar sterile powder, active ingredients of, 248
Ticarcillin, antibacterials containing, 242
 for otitis externa, 108
 ototoxicity of, 149*t*
Ticks, ceruminous otitis caused by, 194
 ear disorders caused by, 92–94, *94*
Tobradex Suspension, active ingredients of, 248
Tobramycin, antibacterials containing, 242
 ototoxicity of, 147*t*
Tolnaftate, as safe ototopical agent, 153*t*
Toluene, ototoxicity of, 149*t*
Tomcat catheter, for cleaning ear canal, 35, *36*
 for tympanic membrane assessment, 38
 in myringotomy, *39,* 39–40

Topagen Ointment, active ingredients of, 248

Topical therapy. See also *Ototopical agents.*
overuse of, otitis externa caused by, 55
tympanic membrane perforation and, 146, 148–153

Toy Poodle, with chronic otitis media, eardrum rupture in, *37*

Tragus, *2, 4,* 5

Trauma, to ear canal, 62–67
from cotton-tipped applicators, 64–66, *65–66,* 105, *171*
from instrumentation, 66–67, *67,* 196
surgical, 62–64

Tresaderm, active ingredients of, 248

Triamcinolone, as safe ototopical agent, 153*t*

Triamcinolone acetonide, products containing, 240

Trichoepithelioma, of ear canal, 195

Triethanolamine, ototoxicity of, 149*t*

Triethyl tin bromide, ototoxicity of, 149*t*

Trigeminal nerve. See *Cranial nerve V (trigeminal).*

Trimethyl tin chloride, ototoxicity of, 149*t*

Tri-Otic, active ingredients of, 248

TrisEDTA. See *EDTA-Tris.*

Tritop, active ingredients of, 248–249

Tubus auris, 5, *5*

Tumor(s). See also *specific tumor.*
interstitial cell, ceruminous otitis with, 186
mast cell, of ear canal, 195
of ear canal, 67–78
benign, 75, 195
biopsy of, 72–74, *74, 76–77*
ceruminous otitis caused by, 195–196
clinical signs of, 68–72, 195–196
diagnosis of, 196
differential diagnosis of, 68, *71–72,* 196
gross examination of, 72–78, *73–74, 76–77*
histopathology of, *72,* 72–74, 78
in cats, 75, 195
in dogs, 75, 195
incidence of, 75
infection associated with, 68–72, *70*
inflammation and, 74–75
localization of, 75
malignant, 75, 195
obscured by wax, 68, *69*
pathogenesis of, 74–75
radiation therapy for, 78
recurrence of, 75
surgical management of, 75–78, 196
treatment of, 75–78, 196
ulcerated, 68, *70*

Tumor(s) *(Continued)*
of middle ear, 68, *71,* 75
Sertoli cell, ceruminous otitis with, 186

Tympanic bulla, *28*
anatomy of, 16–18, *19,* 125–126, 132, *133*
computed tomography of, 132
flushing of, in otitis media, *136–138,* 136–139
flushing solution in, radiographic appearance of, 132, *135*
imaging of, 198–199
in otitis media, 122
inflammatory polyps in, 80
new bone production or remodeling in, 132, *134*
osseous, structure of, *10,* 12–14, *13–15*
otoscopic appearance of, 138, *138*
pathology of, otoscopic findings in, *38,* 38–39
radiographic assessment of, 131–132, *133–135*
factors affecting, 132
with neoplasia, 68, *71*
resection of, in otitis media, 142
suctioning of, 136–138, *137*

Tympanic cavity, *7,* 126

Tympanic membrane, *28*
anatomy of, *7,* 9–12, *10–11, 14,* 125–126
assessment of, *37,* 37–39, *38,* 105, 123, *124,* 125, 148–150, 170, *170*
ceruminolith removal and, 161–164, *163–166*
color of, change in, *38,* 38–39
examination of, 29–32, *30–31,* 123–125, 231
healing of, *173,* 173–178
cytology of, 173–174
otitis media and, 138, 140, *141,* 141–142, 174–178, *175–176*
vascular component of, *173,* 173–174
histology of, 11–12, 125–126, *126,* 156
innervation of, 8
integrity of, assessment of, *38,* 105, 123, *124,* 125, 148–150, 170, *170*
limbus of, *19*
otoscopic appearance of, 29–32, *30–31*
pars flaccida of, 9–10, *11,* 173, *173*
otoscopic appearance of, 30, *30–31*
pars tensa of, 9–11, *11, 19*
otoscopic appearance of, 29, *30*
pathology of, otoscopic findings in, *38,* 38–39
perforation of, permanent, *137, 177,* 177–178, *178*
topical therapy and, 131, 146, 148–153
traumatic, 64, *64,* 65, *66,* 67, *67,* 170–171, *171*
rupture of, 129–130, *129–130*
causes of, 170–173

Tympanic membrane *(Continued)*
  chronic otitis externa and, *101,* 104–106
  chronic otitis media and, 37, *37*
  diagnosis of, 125
  ear mites and, 90, *91,* 157, *158*
  flushing of ear canal and, 32–33, 104–105, 125
  healing of, *173,* 173–178
  inflammatory polyps and, 80–81, 171–173, *172*
  positive contrast radiography in, 125
  sneezing-induced, in cats, 171, *172*
  topical therapy and, 146, 148–153
  traumatic, 64, *64*
  shape of, change in, *38,* 38–39
  tears in, *136*
    after ceruminolith removal, 161–164, *165–166*
  umbo of, 11, *11*
  vasculature of, 12, 30, *31*
Tympanic nerve, *15,* 18–19
  injury to, 19
Tympanic plexus, *15,* 18
Tympanic reflex, 16
Tympano-occipital fissure, 13

U
Umbo, of tympanic membrane, 11, *11*
Utricle, *14,* 22
Utricular nerve, *20–21*

V
Vagus nerve. See *Cranial nerve X (vagus).*
Vancomycin, ototoxicity of, 149*t*
Vascular strip, of eardrum, 30, *31,* 173, *173*
Vestibular ganglion, *20–21*
Vestibular membrane, *20–21,* 22
Vestibular nerve, *19, 20–21*
Vestibular (oval) window, 12, *13,* 14, *14,* 15–16
Vestibule, 16, 20, 22. See also *Saccule; Utricle.*
  ototoxins and, 131
Vestibulocochlear nerve. See *Cranial nerve VIII (acoustic).*
Video Vetscope, 33–37, *34, 36*
  advantages of, 230
  ceruminolith removal using, 161, *163*
  ear mite visualization using, 88
  eardrum rupture diagnosis using, 125
  foreign body removal using, 97
  in staff education, 229
  inflammatory polyp removal using, 83–85, *84*

Video Vetscope *(Continued)*
  inflammatory polyp visualization using, 81, *82*
  tumor removal using, 78
  tumor visualization using, 68
  tympanic membrane suctioning using, 136–138, *137*
Vinblastine, ototoxicity of, 147*t*
Vincristine, ototoxicity of, 147*t*
Viomycin, ototoxicity of, 149*t*
Vitamin A, biological functions of, 188
  metabolism of, in cats, 188
  supplementation of, 188
Vitamin A–responsive dermatosis, ceruminous otitis in, 188
  clinical signs of, 188
  diagnosis of, 188
  treatment of, 188
Vitamin C supplements, 216
Vitamin E supplements, 216
Vomiting, ear canal irritation and, 9
VoSol HC Otic, active ingredients of, 249

W
Water Pik, use of, 105
West Highland white terrier, epidermal dysplasia of, 183
  primary idiopathic seborrhea in, 183
Whipworm, treatment of, 218
Wound(s), facial, and communication with ear canal, 62, *63*
  of ear canal, 62–64, *63–64*

Y
Yeast(s). See also *Malassezia.*
  colonization of ear canal by, in otitis externa, *44,* 106–107
  in ceruminous otitis, 182
  microscopic detection of, 41, *42–43*
  otitis externa caused by, cytological evaluation for, 102–104, *103*
    treatment of, 61–62
  otitis media caused by, treatment of, 140
Yorkshire terrier, otitis externa in, *47*

Z
Zepp lateral ear resection, postoperative complications of, 64
Zinc, supplementation of, 189, 216
Zinc undecylenate, antifungals containing, 243
Zinc-responsive dermatosis, ceruminous otitis with, 188–189
Zygomaticus muscle, *3*

ISBN 0-7216-7750-9

90071